# Congenital Cystic Lung Disease

Haruhiko Sago • Hiroomi Okuyama
Yutaka Kanamori
Editors

# Congenital Cystic Lung Disease

## Comprehensive Understanding of its Diagnosis and Treatment from Fetus to Childhood

Springer

*Editors*
Haruhiko Sago
Center for Maternal-Fetal, Neonatal and Reproductive Medicine
National Center for Child Health and Development
Okura, Setagaya-ku
Tokyo
Japan

Hiroomi Okuyama
Department of Pediatric Surgery
Osaka University Graduate School of Medicine
Yamadaoka, Suita
Osaka
Japan

Yutaka Kanamori
Division of Surgery
Department of Surgical Specialties
National Center for Child Health and Development
Okura, Setagaya-ku
Tokyo
Japan

ISBN 978-981-15-5177-2 ISBN 978-981-15-5175-8 (eBook)
https://doi.org/10.1007/978-981-15-5175-8



This Springer imprint is published by the registered company Springer Nature Singapore Pte Ltd.
The registered company address is: 152 Beach Road, #21-01/04 Gateway East, Singapore 189721, Singapore

# Preface

“Congenital cystic lung disease” is a nomenclature indicating maldevelopment of the lungs. Its etiology is attributed to an unknown cause in fetal age and includes some cystic lung diseases with different etiologies, such as congenital pulmonary airway malformation, bronchial atresia, and intra- and extra-lobar pulmonary sequestration. With the progress achieved in diagnostic modalities (i.e., fetal ultrasound and fetal magnetic resonance imaging) in the past few decades, it has become possible to diagnose these lung diseases in fetal life. As a result, medical staff specializing in diverse fields are involved in the management of such diseases. Nowadays, medical staff in the field of fetal, perinatal, and neonatal medicine, as well as pediatric surgeons, pediatric pathologists, and pediatric radiologists, need to participate in the diagnosis and therapy of the disease.

Considering these new aspects, we planned to publish a textbook that reviews the classification, diagnosis, treatment, and long-term prognosis of congenital cystic lung disease. In order to accomplish our purpose, we asked several physicians (i.e., obstetricians, neonatologists, pediatric pulmonologists, pediatric surgeons, pathologists, and radiologists) in Japan to submit a chapter concerning their respective field of expertise. Owing to their valuable efforts, we were able to publish this comprehensive textbook regarding congenital cystic lung disease, with each chapter containing up-to-date and informative content.

Prof. Kuroda presented the novel classification of congenital cystic lung disease, which was recently addressed by a Japanese working group. Prof. Fuchimoto summarized the epidemiology of the disease, and Dr. Sago summarized the fetal diagnosis and fetal treatment. Dr. Miyazaki described fetal imaging in detail, while Dr. Nozawa discussed the postnatal imaging of the disease. Dr. Ito presented the perinatal treatment of the disease, especially the specific care for the most severe cases, and Prof. Watanabe summarized the integrated postnatal natural history and treatment of the disease. Dr. Usui, Prof. Okuyama, Dr. Kanamori, Dr. Mochizuki, and Dr. Maeda described the specific treatment for each subtype of the disease. Prof. Yamataka provided a special comment related to endoscopic surgery, and Dr. Tanaka proposed a novel idea for the classification of congenital cystic lung disease from a pathological standpoint. Lastly, Dr. Tazuke commented on the long-term prognosis of patients who received surgical treatment at a pediatric age.

Through these very broad-based chapters, the reader can access the latest information regarding congenital cystic lung disease. We hope this textbook will be informative and useful for readers who are concerned with the fetal, perinatal, and postnatal care of congenital cystic lung disease worldwide.

Finally, we wish to express our gratitude to all the authors who contributed to this valuable book.

Tokyo, Japan Haruhiko Sago
Osaka, Japan Hiroomi Okuyama
Tokyo, Japan Yutaka Kanamori

# Contents

# 1 Novel Classification of Congenital Cystic Lung Disease

Tatsuo Kuroda

**Abstract**

The classification of congenital cystic lung disease (CCLD) has been confusing for many years, mostly because the clinical entities included in the previous classifications are not independent mutually and there are many overlapping or "hybrid lesion" of the different entities seen in the clinical practice. In order to solve these problems, a novel classification of CCLD was recently proposed in Japan based on the results of the nationwide survey of CCLD, the pathological review, and the systematic review of the literatures. The new classification divides CCLD into five major entities according to the embryology how the lesion is formed during the development of the lung: (1) pulmonary airway malformation; (2) lung bud malformation; (3) foregut malformation; (4) bronchial atresia; and (5) others. To avoid overlapping of each entity of CCLD, the diseases included in each entity are defined only by the lesions primarily formed during the pulmonary development. Thus, the term "hybrid lesion" is abandoned, and the exclusion criteria is prescribed strictly. The present classification redefines each entity of CCLD more clearly and aims to correlate the clinical feature and pathological diagnosis more closely. The novel classification is presented and explained in this chapter.

**Keywords**

Congenital cystic lung disease · Classification Congenital pulmonary airway malformation Lung bud malformation · Bronchopulmonary sequestration · Bronchopulmonary foregut malformation · Foregut malformation Bronchial atresia

## 1.1 Introduction

It is well known that there are several different clinical entities in congenital cystic lung disease (CCLD). However, the classification of CCLD has been unestablished and confusing for many years, although several classifications based on the different backgrounds such as pathology and embryology have been proposed before. A certain population of CCLD patients are known to develop a critical pathophysiology resulting in intrauterine fetal death or respiratory distress immediately after birth. Nevertheless, the clinical features of each entity of CCLD has remained unclear. This is mostly because the respective clinical entities in the previous classifications are not independent mutually and numerous overlapping

T. Kuroda (✉)
Department of Pediatric Surgery, Keio University, School of Medicine, Tokyo, Japan
e-mail: kuroda-t@keio.jp





H. Sago et al. (eds.), *Congenital Cystic Lung Disease*, https://doi.org/10.1007/978-981-15-5175-8_1

cases are consequently seen in the practical clinics, which were often regarded as a "hybrid lesion" of the different entities. The establishment of a clinically more practical and well-defined classification of CCLD is required especially in the era when the prenatal surgical intervention is enabled. The Japanese Study Group of Pediatric Chest Surgery conducted a nationwide survey on CCLD to examine the clinical features of CCLD from the perinatal period through the late postoperative period [1, 2]. Some novel findings to redefine each entity of CCLD were obtained in the survey, thus a newly organized classification of CCLD based on the embryology was proposed by the study group. The present chapter describes this recently proposed classification of CCLD and explains how each entity of CCLD is prescribed more exclusively.

## 1.2 Novel Classification Based on the Embryology

1. Overview (Table 1.1)

   CCLD is defined as the state that a pathological and irreversible cystic lesion except for dilated bronchi exists in the pulmonary parenchyma congenitally. In the previous classifications of CCLD, the pathohistological findings of the lesion primarily formed during the pulmonary development and those findings formed secondarily due to another pulmonary maldevelopment or acquired infection are not distinguished exclusively, which made the definition of each CCLD entity unclear, and produced overlapping of different clinical entities. The new classification divides CCLD into five major entities according to the embryology how the lesion is primarily formed during the development of the lung: (1) pulmonary airway malformation; (2) lung bud malformation; (3) foregut malformation; (4) bronchial atresia; and (5) others. Each entity is defined only by the primary maldevelopment, and the diseases developed secondarily by some other etiology such as vascular anomalies and acquired infection are all excluded from each entity of CCLD.

2. Pulmonary airway malformation

   The most representative entity in CCLD is named as pulmonary airway malformation, which includes diseases resulted from the delay or arrest of pulmonary development from the lung bud. In 1997, Stocker et al. [3] first described this entity of CCLD as congenital cystic adenomatoid malformation (CCAM) based on the pathohistological observation that the cyst wall showed adenomatoid finding. Initially, Stocker and his colleagues presumed that CCAM might be a kind of hamartomatous or neoplastic lesion formed during the lung development. They divided CCAM into three subtypes according to the cyst size; type I contains a macroscopic cyst bigger than 1 cm in diameter, type II does a cyst with 0.5 ~ 1.0 cm in diameter, and type III contains a microcystic lesion with the cyst

**Table 1.1** New classification of congenital cystic lung disease

| | Entity | Diseases included | Exclusion criteria |
|---|---|---|---|
| 1. | Pulmonary airway malformation | • Congenital pulmonary airway malformation (type 0–4) etc. | ✓ accompanying other congenital airway obstructive disease |
| | | | ✓ "hybrid lesion" with a disease of the other entity of CCLD |
| 2. | Lung bud malformation | • Intra-lobar and extra-lobar bronchopulmonary sequestration | ✓ lesion with bronchi directing the normal pulmonary hilum |
| | | • Bronchopulmonary foregut malformation etc. | ✓ lesion without elastic artery originated from the systemic major artery |
| 3. | Foregut malformation | • Bronchogenic cyst etc. | |
| 4. | Bronchial atresia | • Bronchial atresia | |
| 5. | Others | • Lymphangiectasis etc. | |

size less than 0.5 cm in diameter. However, later in 1994, Stocker [4] proposed to change the concept of CCAM from the neoplastic lesion to developmental arrest or delay during the airway and the lung development, and renamed this entity of disease as congenital pulmonary airway malformation (CPAM), which was furthermore revised in 2002 [5]. In his new concept, type 0 and type 4 were added, and previous type I to III of CCAM corresponded to type 1 to 3 of CPAM. Each subtype is defined by the level of airway where the developmental arrest or delay occurs. In type 0, the developmental arrest occurs at the central airway; therefore, no further lung tissue develops subsequently. Then the developmental arrest occurs at the bronchial, bronchiolar, bronchiolar to alveolar, and distal acinar levels in type 1, 2, 3, and 4 CPAM, respectively. The new concept of CPAM has been widely accepted. The present classification also supports Stocker's new proposal, and has introduced this concept and his new classification of CPAM as the first entity of CCLD without major modification.

3. Lung bud malformation

The second entity includes diseases that are considered to develop from the abnormally excessive lung bud, that is, accessory lung bud. Intra- and extra-lobar bronchopulmonary sequestration (BPS) and bronchopulmonary foregut malformation (BPFM) are the representative diseases included in this entity. The sequestrated lung is defined as a lung tissue with no communication with the normal bronchial tree. Intra-lobar BPS is located in the normal lung lobe and shares the common pleural membrane, whereas extra-lobar BPS is located outside of the normal lobe and covered by its proper pleural membrane independently from the normal lobes. Early in 1902, Eppinger [6] had already stated that accessory lung bud might be the etiology to form the sequestrated lung. The modern concept of BPS was first described by Pryce [7] as an intra-lobar or an extra-lobar pulmonary lesion accompanied by one or more aberrant arteries originated from the aorta or the elastic systemic artery. Pryce paid more attention to this aberrant artery rather than the sequestrated lung and supposed that the sequestrated lung lesion might be secondarily formed by the traction of this aberrant artery during pulmonary development. Based on this traction theory, Pryce divided BPS in three subtypes according to the style of the aberrant artery; type 1 has an aberrant artery originated from the systemic circulation but no sequestrated lesion, type 2 has an aberrant artery that infiltrate into the normal lung beyond the sequestrated lung, and type 3 has an aberrant artery that flows limitedly in the sequestrated lung (Fig. 1.1). Later, some cases that were unclassifiable by this classification were reported, and several alterations and modification of Pryce's classification were subsequently proposed until recently [8, 9, 10, 11]. In contrast to the Pryce's traction hypothesis as an etiology of BPS, Ishida and his colleague [12] reported an observation that the bronchial tree in the sequestrated lung point to the identical peripheral site where a single aberrant artery flows into the sequestrated lung in a certain cohort of intra-lobar BPS, and considered that these lesions might be developed from the accessory lung bud located at the peripheral site as Eppinger described. Ishida proposed to regard only these lesions with bronchi pointing to the peripheral direction as the real sequestrated lung. Since this concept has acquired more support in Japan, the present classification redefines BPS as a malformation developed from the accessory lung bud and confined BPS only to the above lesions. Although an elastic aberrant artery (or multiple arteries in some rare cases) originated from the systemic major artery is also an essential morphological feature seen in BPS, the precise classification according to the styles of the aberrant artery no longer has so much impact in the present classification. Therefore, Pryce's classification of BPS is not introduced in the present classification.

On the other hand, a sequestrated lung lesion communicating with the esophagus

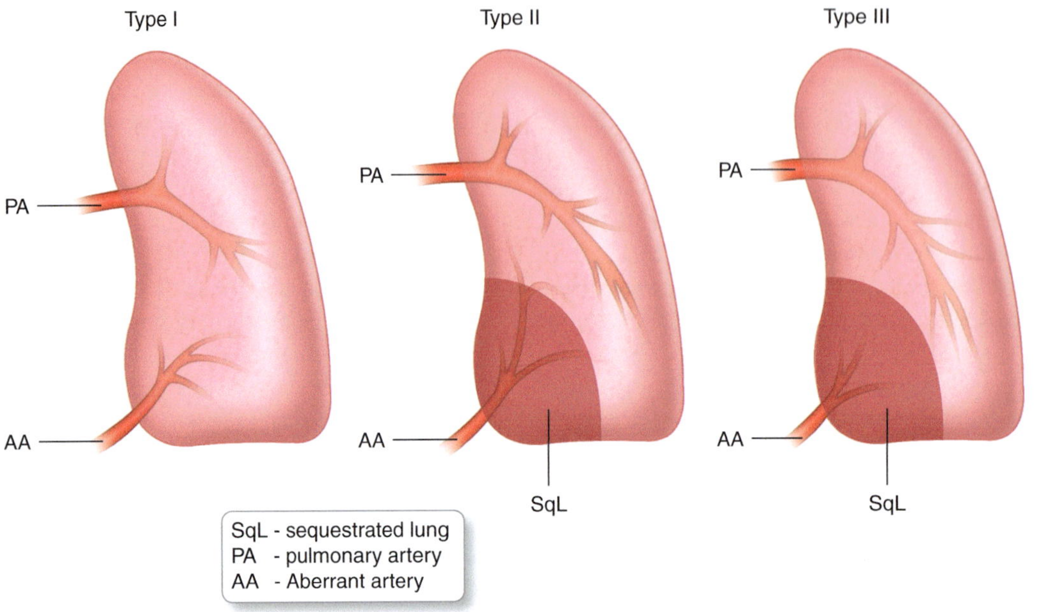


**Fig. 1.1** Pryce's classification of intra-lobar bronchopulmonary sequestration

was first described by Klebs [13] in 1874. The term "BPFM" was first described by Gerle [14] et al. in 1968. In their initial report, BPFM was defined by intra- or extra-lobar BPS sometimes accompanied by bronchial communication with the gastrointestinal tract and also by diaphragmatic hernia. More recently, Morikawa et al. [15] reviewed the origin of the artery in the lesion in their own series and also in the literatures, and redefined BPFM as a sequestrated lung accompanied by the bronchi originated from the gastrointestinal tract. Then he concluded that BPFM also developed from the accessory lung bud. The present classification supports this concept, and recognizes BPFM as a special subtype of BPS.

4. Foregut malformation

The third entity includes the lesions formed by the abnormal development of the foregut. Bronchogenic cysts are located adhesively to the central airway or the esophagus. These lesions are considered to be formed by the abnormal division of the foregut in the present classification.

5. Bronchial atresia

Atresia at the various levels of the airway forms the cystic lesion in the distal lung parenchyma of the atretic bronchi or bronchiole. In addition, bronchial atresia shows a variety of pathological features such as emphysema, atelectasis, obstructive pneumonia, and bronchial mucocele [16, 17]. Some of the pathohistological findings seen in bronchial atresia seem extremely similar to those seen in CPAM type 2 [17]. Therefore, previously, a considerable number of patients with bronchia atresia might have been diagnosed as having CPAM. On the other hand, it has been questionable whether bronchial atresia should be regarded as one of CCLD or not. Abnormal origin of bronchi with atresia due to the anomaly of pulmonary artery was observed especially in the left upper lobe [18]. In these cases, bronchial atresia may not be a primary maldevelopment but a secondarily lesion developed in association with the vascular anomaly, which may not meet the inclusion criteria of CCLD. However, it is proposed to include bronchial atresia as one of the entities of CCLD in the present classification, because there are so many shared pathological findings between other entities of CCLD and bronchial atresia; therefore, the concept to include bronchial atresia into CCLD seems more convenient from the perspective of differential diagnosis.

6. Others

   Other congenital cystic lesions of the lung such as congenital pulmonary lymphangiectasis are included in this entity.

## 1.3 Pathology Secondary to Lung Maldevelopment

It has been a major problem in terms of the classification of CCLD that there exists an overlap of the different entities. The term "hybrid lesion" has been often used for the cases that show both of CPAM-like and non-CPAM-like findings in a single lesion. Langston [19] proposed to classify the CCLDs into the distinct pathological entities in his review in 2003. According to our nationwide survey of CCLD [1, 2], CPAM is more obviously associated with the critical perinatal features such as fetal hydrops and respiratory distress immediately after birth when compared with other entities of CCLD such as bronchial atresia and bronchopulmonary sequestration. Furthermore, in some literatures including our own, the larger volume of the fetal lung lesion is associated with the more critical features [2, 20]. Nevertheless, lesion volume index measured during the fetal period did not show the significant difference between the patients diagnosed to have CPAM and those who were diagnosed to have non-CPAM lesions in our survey [2]. This paradoxical observation may be explained by the overlapped diagnosis of CPAM and non-CPAM entities. There may be a possibility that a considerable portion of these cases have been misdiagnosed as CPAM, instead of other less critical diseases such as bronchial atresia or BPS. Langston [19] insisted that some of the CPAM type 2-like lesion should be regarded as the secondary malformation sequence based on airway obstruction rather than the hybrid lesion of two different entities of fetal lung malformations, and demonstrated two types of CPAM type 2-like findings as the malformation sequence: (1) parenchymal maldevelopment of the pulmonary hyperplasia and (2) microcystic parenchymal maldevelopment. Takakuwa, Nakazawa and their colleagues [17, 21] also supported Langston's new concept according to their observations in a Japanese series. They examined the pathohistology of bronchial atresia cases, and observed that microcystic parenchymal maldevelopment, a highly CPAM type 2-like lesion, was observed in 37.5% of the bronchial atresia cases, whereas parenchymal maldevelopment of the pulmonary hyperplasia was observed in 90.9% among them. These findings should not be regarded as the feature specifically indicating the diagnosis of CPAM. Instead, they should be recognized as the pathological features suggesting of bronchial atresia. Thus, it is highly insisted in the present classification of CCLD that the term "hybrid lesion" should be abandoned.

## 1.4 Precise Definition of Each Entity of CCLD and Exclusion of the Unfit Lesions

In addition to abrogation of the term "hybrid lesion," some proposals are made to define the diseases included in each entity of CCLD more clearly and exclude unmet cases in the present classification.

1. Lobar emphysema

   Historically, lobar emphysema was considered as one of the CCLD entities. However, it has been pointed out that lobar emphysema is observed in many entities of CCLD such as bronchial atresia. Nowadays, lobar emphysema is not regarded as an independent clinical entity but a clinical symptom secondary to airway obstruction. Unlike the emphysema in adult, the wall of air spaces is not irreversibly destroyed in lobar emphysema seen in childhood; therefore, lobar emphysema is considered to be a reversible manifestation due to an obstructive mechanism of the airway.

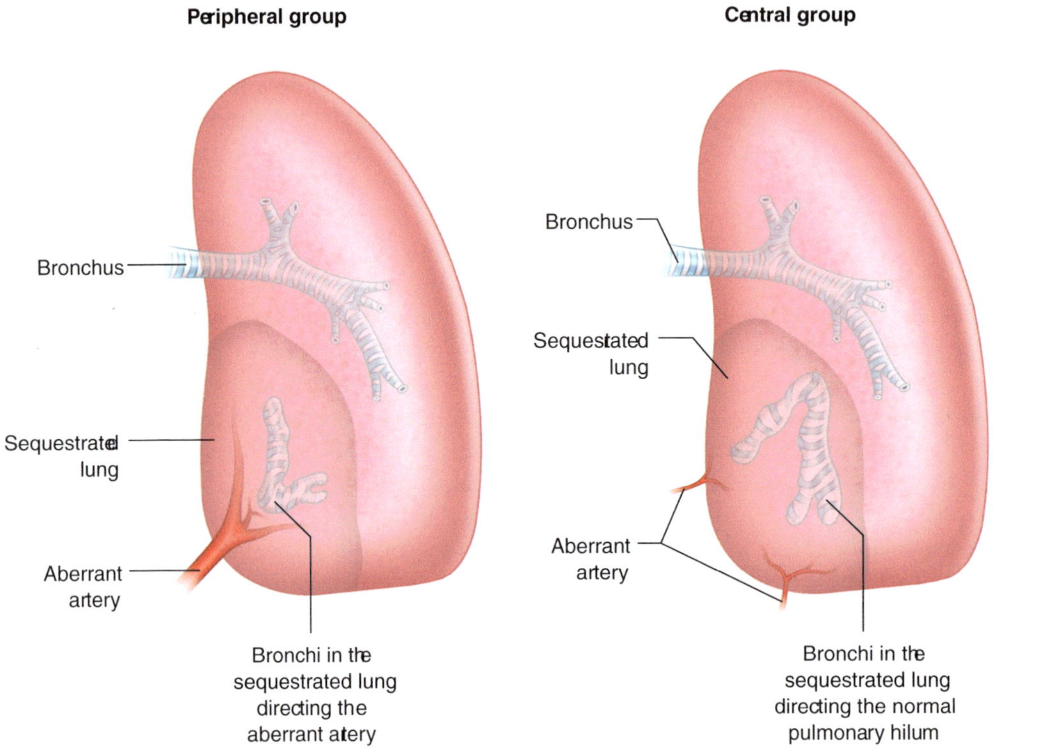


**Fig. 1.2** The peripheral and the central groups in previously called "intra-lobar bronchopulmonary sequestration"

2. Vascular hyperplasia and the aberrant artery in bronchopulmonary sequestration (BPS) (Fig. 1.2.)

   Ishida and his colleagues [12, 22] reviewed the macroscopic pathology of the patients that was once diagnosed as having intra-lobar BPS. They observed that these patients could be divided into two different groups according to the direction of bronchi and the vascular findings in the lesion: the central group and the peripheral group. In the central group, bronchi in the lesion point to the normal pulmonary hilum and multiple and fine aberrant arteries are accompanied, whereas in the peripheral group, bronchi point to the peripheral region where the single elastic aberrant artery flows into the lesion. The formation of the lesion in the peripheral group is well explained by the excessive accessory lung bud embryologically. Therefore, only these lesions of the peripheral group are recognized as BPS in the present classification as cited above. On the other hand, Kamagata et al. [22] estimated that the multiple small arteries seen in the lesions of the central group are not the primary aberrant arteries but secondary vascular hyperplasia due to infection. Kamagata's observation and the direction of bronchi in the lesion indicated that those lesions of the central group are considered to be formed due to bronchial atresia and modified by acquired infection. For this reason, the lesions of the central group are excluded from BPS in the present classification.

3. Abnormal origin of the pulmonary artery

   In the present classification, the sequestrated lung is considered as the pulmonary tissue developed from the accessory lung bud unlike the initial concept of BPS described by Pryce in 1946 [7]. Although Pryce's classification [7] of intra-lobar BPS has been the gold standard, aberrant artery flows into the normal lung lobe that has no sequestrated lung tissue in his type 1 BPS. According to the change of the key feature defining BPS from the aberrant artery to the sequestrated lung tissue developed from the accessory lung bud, type 1 subgroup of Pryce's classification can no longer be regarded as bronchopulmonary sequestration in the present classification. In the present classification, these lesions are considered as an abnormal origin of the pulmonary artery, which is not a lung maldevelopment but a vascular malformation [12, 23], and excluded from CCLD.

4. Abnormal origin of the bronchi

   The definition of bronchopulmonary foregut malformation (BPFM) remains also unestablished. Lung lesion with bronchi originated from gastrointestinal tract such as the esophagus was widely called BPFM in the previous literatures. Morikawa et al. [15] observed that there are two different types of lesions in so called "BPFM"; the lesions fed by normal pulmonary artery, and those fed by an artery originated from the aorta (Fig. 1.3). The former lesions have no sequestrated lung developed from the accessory lung bud. Therefore, the present classification confined BPFM only to the latter type of the lesions, and excluded the former lesions from BPFM. These lesions without the sequestrated lung are regarded as the mal-origin of bronchi instead of pulmonary maldevelopment.

## 1.5 Future Aspect of the Novel Classification

As stated above, the retrospective analysis based on the previous classification failed to show the statistically significant difference between CPAM and non-CPAM cases in our survey [2], though many clinical observations suggested that the clinical feature of CPAM seemed quite different from that of non-CPAM diseases. The clinical features of each entities of CCLD have been uncleared because of overlapping of diagnosis due to the ambiguity of the classification. The present classification redefines CPAM more

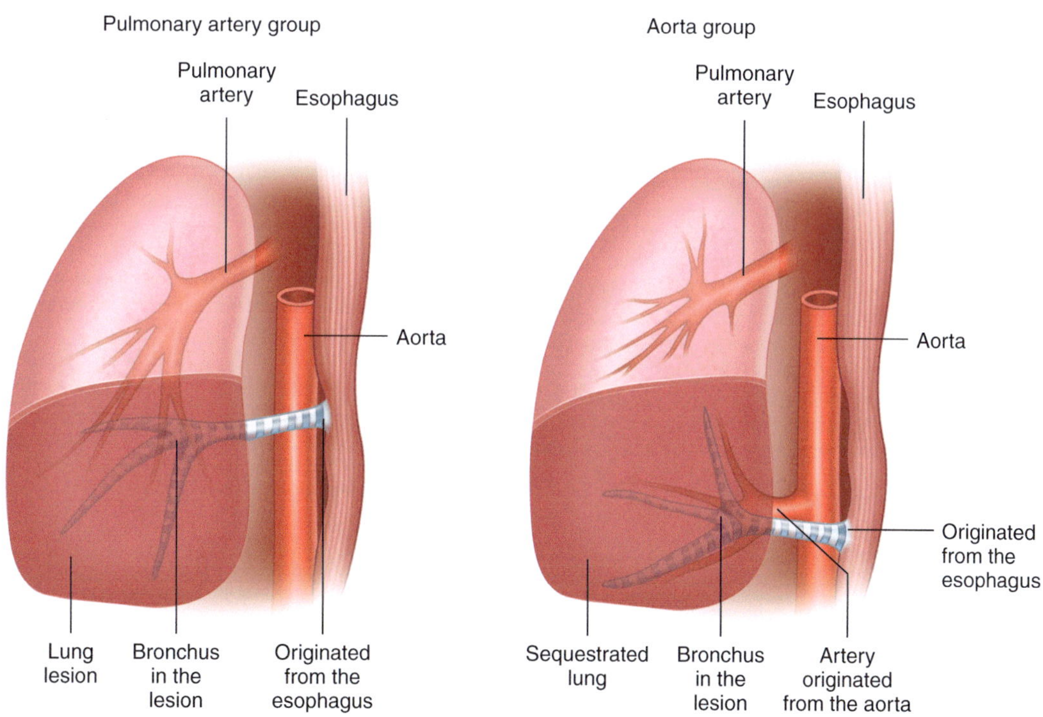


**Fig. 1.3** Two different groups in previously called BPFM

strictly and aims to exclude non-CPAM lesions from this entity. Due to these revisions, the novel classification is expected to clear the true clinical features in each clinical entity of CCLD. The association between clinical features and the embryology of the lung maldevelopment may be cleared also in the future. The precise diagnosis based on the proper classification may indicate the most suitable treatment strategy including prenatal surgical intervention for each clinical entity of CCLD. The novel classification is expected to be more useful in the clinical practice compared to before. The pathological review of the past cases based on the novel classification should be also required to verify the efficacy of the present classification in the future studies.

## References

1. Kuroda T, Nishijima E, Maeda K, et al. Clinical features of congenital cystic lung diseases; a report on a nationwide multicenter study in Japan. European J Pediatr Surg. 2016;26:91–5.
2. Kuroda T, Nishijima E, Maeda K, et al. Perinatal features of congenital cystic lung diseases: results of a nationwide multicentric study in Japan. Pediatr Surg Int. 2016;32(9):827–31.
3. Stocker JT, Madewell JE, Drake RM. Congenital cystic adenomatoid malformation of the lung. Hum Pathol. 1977;8:155–71.
4. Stocker JT. Congenital and developmental diseases. In: Dail DH, Sp H, editors. Pulmonary pathology (Ed 2). New York: NY, Springer-Verlag; 1944. p. 174–80.
5. Stocker JT. Congenital pulmonary airway malformation – a new name for and an expanded classification of congenital cystic adenomatoid malformation of the lung. Histopathology. 2002;41(suppl, 2):424–30.
6. Eppinger H, Sauenstein W (1902) Krankheiten der Lungen Ergeb Alleg Path 8:267–365.
7. Pryce DM. Lower accessory pulmonary artery with intralobar sequestration of lung; a report of seven cases. J Pathol Bact. 1946;58:457–67.
8. Sade RM, Clouse M, Ellis FH. Spectrum of pulmonary sequestration. Ann Thorc Surg. 1974;18:644–58.
9. Flye MW, Conley M, Silver D. The spectrum of pulmonary sequestration. Ann Thorc Surg. 1976;22:478–82.
10. Thilenius OG, Ruschhaupt DG, Replogle RL, et al. Spectrum of pulmonary sequestration. Association with anomalous pulmonary venous drainage in infants. Ped Cardiolo. 1983;4:97–103.
11. Shindo G, Iwai W, Yoneda R, et al. Clinicopathological analysis of 12 cases with intralobar pulmonary sequestration – with focusing on the pathological study in the etiology. Jpn J Chest Dis. 1973;32:9–22.
12. Ishida H, Hajikano H, Hayashi A. Intralobar sequestrationin children- a new concept from the form of bronchial tree in sequestrated lung. Jpn J Thorac Cardiovasc Surg. 1992;40:957–68.
13. Klebs E. Missbildungen der Lunge. Aetlt Cor-blf Bohem. 1874;2:111–21.
14. Gerle RD, Jaretzki A, Ashley CA, et al. Congenital bronchopulmonary foregut malformation. New Engl J Med. 1968;278:1413–9.
15. Morikawa N, Ishida H, Hayashi A, et al. A case of bronchopulmonary foregut malformation and its new classification based on blood supply an bronchial findings. J Jpn Soc Pediatr Surg. 1992;28:932–9.
16. Morikawa N, Kuroda T, Honna T, et al. Congenital bronchial atresia in infants and children. J Pediatr Surg. 2005;40:1822–6.
17. Takakuwa E, Iwafuchi H, Hamazaki Y. Pathohistology of bronchial atresia; differential diagnosis from CCAM. Jpn J Pediatr Surg. 2011;43:1273–6.
18. Ishida H. The general concept of congenital pulmonary cystic diseases. Jpn J Chest Dis. 2000;59:81–90.
19. Langston C. New concepts in the pathology of congenital lung malformations. Seminar Pediatr Surg. 2003;12:17–37.
20. Crombleholme TM, Coleman B, Hedrick H, et al. Cystic adenomatoid malformation volume ratio predicts outcome in prenatally diagnosed cystic adenomatoid malformation of the lung. J Pediatr Surg. 2002;37:331–8.
21. Nakazawa A, Matsuoka K, Takakuwa E, et al. A clinicopathological review of the 33 cases with bronchial atresia. J Jpn Soc Pediatr Surg. 2012;48:800.
22. Kamagata S, Ishida H, Hayashi A, et al. Systemic-pulmonary shunt in a patient with pulmonary infection. J Jpn Soc Pediatr Surg. 1993;29:1039–43.
23. Ishida H, Hayashi A, Kamagata S, et al. Basic and new concept of pulmonary sequestration. Jpn J Pediatr Surg. 1993;25:1231–9.

# 2 Epidemiology of Congenital Cystic Lung Disease: From Japan Nationwide Survey

Yasushi Fuchimoto

**Abstract**

We conducted a retrospective study on 428 patients (194 prenatally diagnosed and 234 postnatally diagnosed) with cystic lung diseases who were treated at high-volume facilities in Japan between 1992 and 2012. In 194 prenatally diagnosed cases, thoracic abnormalities were identified by fetal ultrasonographic examination between 12 and 42 weeks of gestation (median: 24 weeks). The ratio (LVR) of fetal pulmonary lesion volume to head circumference was measured in 59 patients, and we observed a decreasing trend in LVR in the third trimester of pregnancy. However, LVR at initial measurement was significantly higher (2.04 ± 1.71 vs 0.98 ± 0.50, $P < 0.00071$) in patients who presented postnatal respiratory symptoms than in asymptomatic patients. Additionally, LVR at initial measurement was significantly higher (2.34 ± 1.79 vs. O.96 ± 0.46, $P < 0.00005$) in patients with fetal hydrops than in those without. Examining the relationship between LVR and pathological diagnosis, we found that patients with CPAM tended to have a higher LVR than patients with non-CPAM disease.

After birth, 12.4% of patients required endotracheal intubation. At postnatal day 30, 67.9% were asymptomatic, but 14% required respiratory support, and 3.3% had died. On the other hand, of patients who were asymptomatic immediately after birth, 33.6% presented symptoms such as respiratory infection in the first year of life, and the cumulative incidence of respiratory symptoms increased to 74.3% at 3 years of age.

No cases of the malignant transformation associated with congenital cystic lung disease were observed in this study.

**Keywords**

Nationwide survey · Epidemiology · Fetal diagnosis · LVR

This nationwide cohort study retrospectively collected data of patients with congenital cystic lung disease (CCLD), who were treated at any of the 10 high-volume centers in Japan between January 1992 and December 2012. A total of 428 patients (194 prenatally diagnosed and 234 postnatally diagnosed) were involved in this study. The demographic data is summarized in Table 2.1. The medical records during the neonatal period were available for 243 patients, including for prenatally and postnatally diagnosed cases.

Y. Fuchimoto (✉)
Department of Pediatric Surgery, International University of Health and Welfare School of Medicine, Chiba, Japan
e-mail: yfuchimoto@iuhw.ac.jp


H. Sago et al. (eds.), *Congenital Cystic Lung Disease*, https://doi.org/10.1007/978-981-15-5175-8_2

**Table 2.1** The demographic data

| | All | Prenatally diagnosed | Postnatally diagnosed | |
|---|---|---|---|---|
| Gender male/female | 224/204 | 103/91 | 121/113 | N.S. |
| Gestational week | 26–43 median 38 | 26–41 median 38 | 26–43 median 38 | N.S. |
| Birth weight (g) | 472–4300 median 2960 | 818–4300 median 2965 | 472–4266 median 2956 | N.S. |
| Birth height (cm) | 29.4–54.0 median 48.8 | 30.0–54.0 median 48.8 | 29.4–52.5 median 48.0 | N.S. |

*N.S.* not significant

**Table 2.2** Prenatal fetal images:fetal ultrasonography and fetal MRI

| Fetal ultrasonography ($n$ = 194) | |
|---|---|
| Space-occupying lesion | 89.20% |
| Hydramnios | 13.60% |
| Mediastinal shift | 51.90% |
| Hydropic signs | 15.20% |
| LHR | 1.1–3.8 (median 1.3) |
| Fetal MRI ($n$ = 96) | |
| Mediastinal shift | 60.60% |
| Fetal hydrops | 9.70% |
| Other hydropic signs | 17.60% |
| Macrocystic | 62.50% |
| Microcystic | 31.20% |

The relevant clinical courses, pre- and postnatal radiological images, risk assessment pathological images, late respiratory function, and complications were retrospectively reviewed after receiving IRB approval from each of the centers. Furthermore, the late postoperative respiratory function was assessed using spirometry in 22 patients after the age of 6 years, which corresponds to the age of the completion of rapid growth in lung development.

## 2.1 Perinatal Clinical Features

### Prenatal

- **Fetal images**

  During fetal exploration of 163 patients using ultrasonography, a space-occupying lesion in the lung was identified in 89.2% of the patients at the time of the initial diagnosis. Accompanying findings included hydramnios in 14.0%, a mediastinal shift in 51.9%, and hydropic signs in 13.6% of patients. The lung head ratio (LHR) ranged from 1.1 to 3.8 (median 1.3) (Table 2.2).

  Fetal MRI was performed during the third trimester in 96 patients. According to the fetal MRI, a mediastinal shift was seen in 60.6% and fetal hydrops was seen in 9.7% of patients. Regarding other hydropic findings, fetal subcutaneous edema, pleural effusion, and ascites were seen in 5.3, 4.4, and 8.8%, of patients, respectively. Macrocystic lesions accounted for 62.5% of the whole cystic lung abnormalities, whereas microcystic lesion accounted for 31.2% from the MRI images (Table 2.2).

- **Prenatal intervention**

  Information regarding prenatal interventions was available for 221 out of 428 neonatal patients. The maternal administration of steroids was prescribed for 18 patients (8.1%), whereas the aspiration of the fetal lung cyst was performed in 23 patients (10.4%), among whom a pleuro-amniotic shunt tube was inserted and placed in 20 patients (9.0%). No prenatal intervention was given to the rest of the patients.

- **Delivery, neonatal findings, and associated abnormalities**

  The delivery modes of 347 patients were natural transvaginal delivery in 49.8%, planned transvaginal delivery in 13.5%, planned caesarean section in 20.1%, emergency caesarean section in 16.6% of cases.

  Regarding the respiratory state immediately after birth, retractive breathing and tachypnea were observed in 29.8% and 29.1% of the neonates, respectively. The APGAR score at 1 min was 8–9 in 75.4%, 6–7 in 11.8%, 4–5 in 6.2%, 1–3 in 6.6% of the patients. Associated malformations were seen in 13.0% of the patients including major cardiovascular abnormalities, congenital diaphragmatic hernia, and renal and urogenital malformation.

- **Risk assessment by fetal ultrasonography: fetal lung lesion volume ratio**

  The fetal lung lesion volume ratio (LVR) measured at the time of the initial diagnosis was significantly higher among the patients who were symptomatic and required hospitalization or respiratory treatment as of postnatal day 30 compared with the asymptomatic patients (2.04 ± 1.71 vs. 0.98 ± 0.50, $P < 0.00071$) (Fig. 2.1). The LVR measured during the late gestational period was higher in the symptomatic patients compared with that of asymptomatic patients; however, the difference was not statistically significant (1.39 ± 1.00 vs. 0.72 ± 0.54). Both, the LVR measured at the time of the initial diagnosis and during the late gestational period were significantly higher among patients who developed fetal hydrops than among those who did not (2.34 ± 1.79 vs. 0.96 ± 0.46, $P < 0.00005$ for initial measurement; 1.61 ± 1.20 vs. 0.78 ± 0.60, $P < 0.048$ for late gestational measurements) (Fig. 2.2). Furthermore, the LVR decreased to a greater degree during the late gestational period in the non-CCAM patients compared with the CCAM patients (from 1.37 ± 1.28 to 1.14 ± 0.84 for the CCAM patients, and from 1.08 ± 0.47 to 0.46 ± 0.64 for the non-CCAM patients), although the difference was not statistically significant (Fig. 2.3).

  On postnatal day 30, a total of 165 of the 243 neonatal patients (67.9%) were asymp-

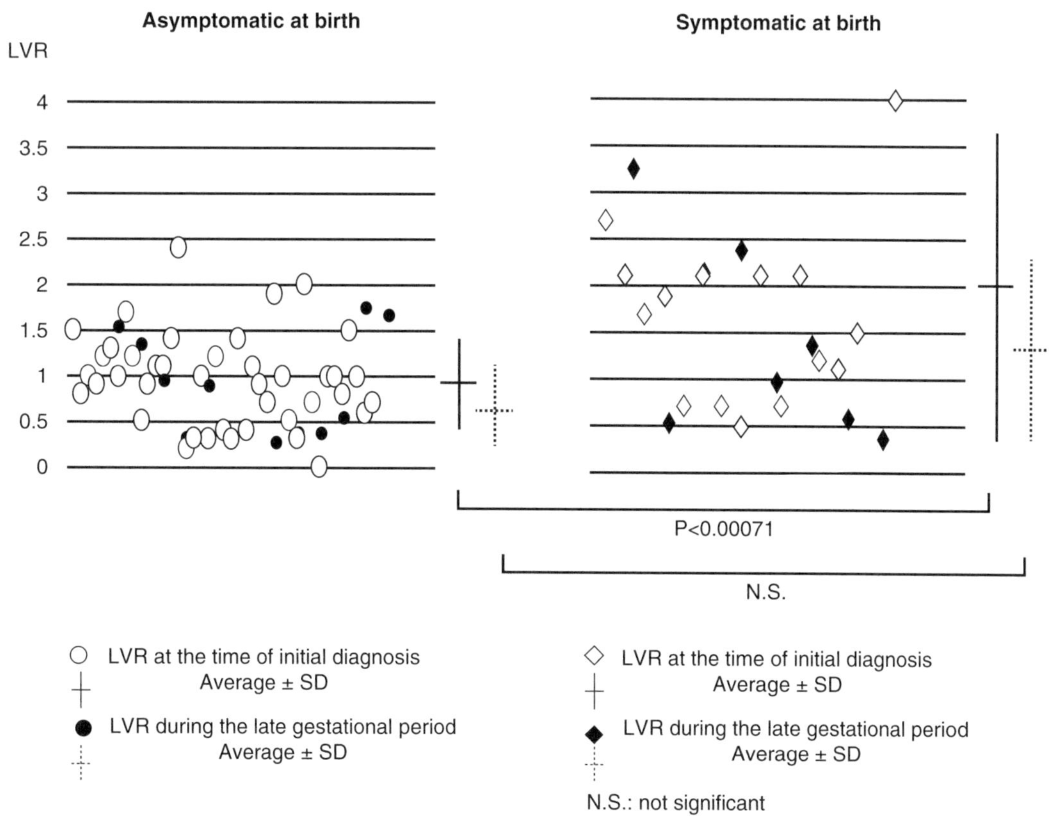


**Fig. 2.1** Association between LVR and clinical outcome. The open marks represent the LVRs measured at the time of the initial diagnosis, and the closed marks represent the LVRs measured during the late gestational period. The bars on the right side of the graph visualize the average and standard deviation of the LVR. The LVR measured at the time of the initial diagnosis was significantly higher among the patients who required hospitalization or respiratory treatment as of postnatal day 30, compared to the asymptomatic patients

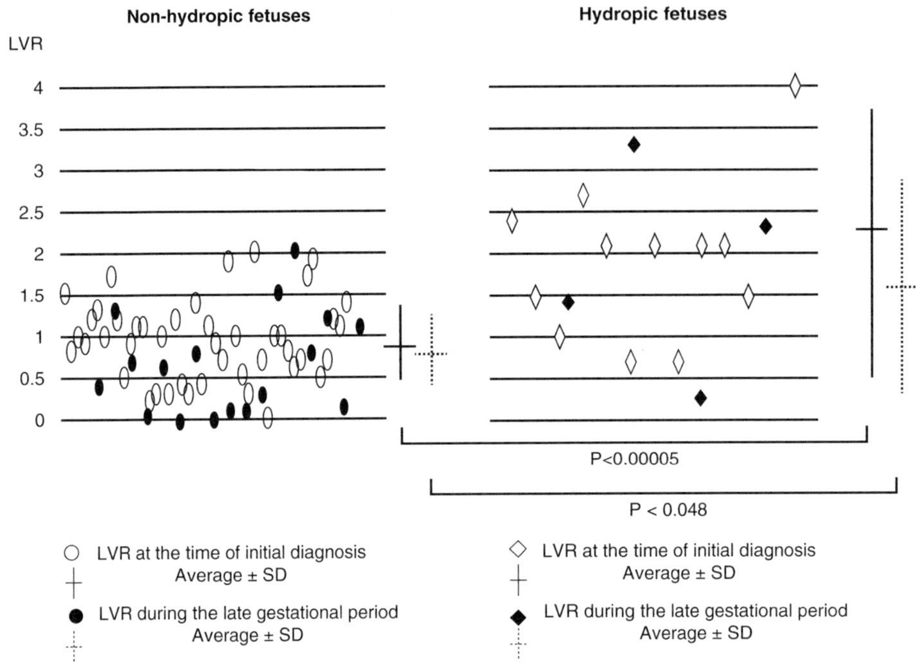


**Fig. 2.2** Association between LVR and fetal hydrops. Both the LVR measured at the time of the initial diagnosis and during the late gestational period were significantly higher among the patients who developed fetal hydrops than those who did not

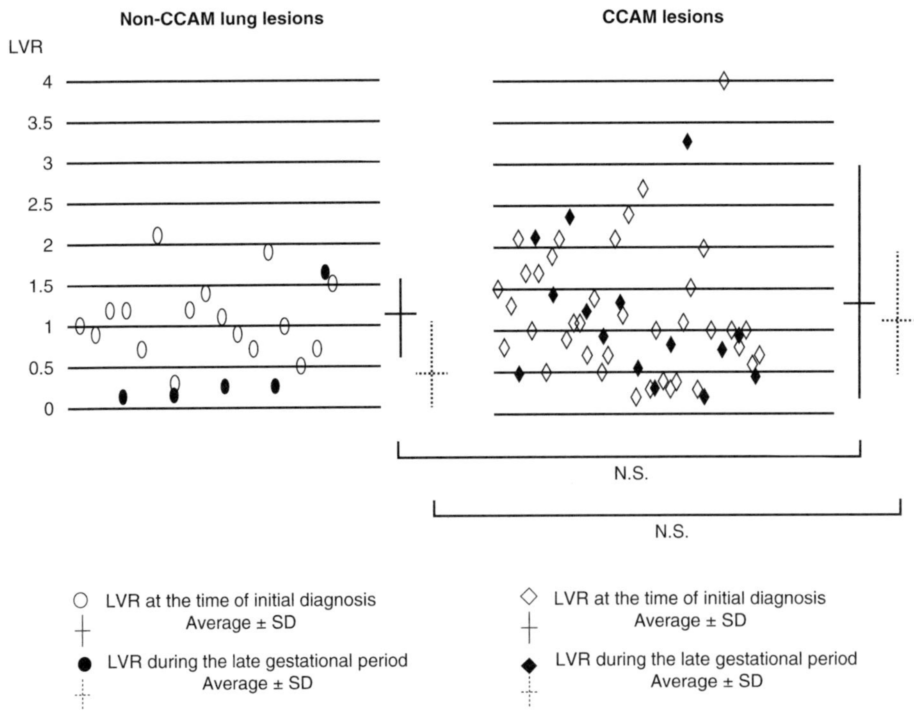


**Fig. 2.3** Association between LVR and pathological diagnosis. The LVR decreased to a greater degree during the late gestational period in the non-CCAM patients, compared with the CCAM patients

tomatic and living at home, 64 (26.3%) required hospitalization, 7 (2.9%) had been transferred to a regional hospital, and 8 (3.3%) died. Thirty-three patients (13.6%) continue to require respiratory treatment including 18 who required the use of a respirator and 6 who required a pulmonary vasodilator. One patient received a tracheotomy. Surgery was performed in 137 patients and was scheduled for 60 patients, whereas 31 patients were under observation without surgery. In one patient, the lung lesion had become unrecognizable.

## 2.2 Later Onset of Clinical Symptoms in Asymptomatic Neonates

Among the patients who were immediately asymptomatic after birth, 140 patients were confirmed to have developed respiratory symptoms after the age of 1 month. Out of those patients, 47 (33.6%) developed pulmonary symptoms within the first year of life. Thereafter, the onset of clinical symptoms was recognized between the age of 1 and 2 years in 31 patients (22.1%). As shown in Fig. 2.4, the cumulated incidence of symptoms related to CCLD drastically increased before the age of 2 years and was 74.3% at the age of 3 years. Only 10 patients (7.1%) developed symptoms after the age of 6 years.

Fever and coughing were the most common initial symptoms seen in 95 patients (67.9%) and 75 patients (53.6%), respectively. Other relatively common symptoms include continuous expectoration of sputum in 9 (6.4%) and chest pain in 8 (5.7%) patients, respectively. A total of 74.0% of the patients exhibited infectious features of the lower airway.

## 2.3 Surgery, Complications, and Clinical Outcome

Out of the 428 patients, 409 patients had undergone surgery at the time of the survey. In 34.8% of these patients, surgery was required due to respiratory symptoms. The surgical procedure performed for CCLD was a monolobectomy in 292 patients (71.4%), a multiple lobectomy in 13 patients (3.2%), a segmentectomy in 32 patients (7.8%), a pneumonectomy in 13 patients (3.2%), and other procedures such as wedge resection and fenestration of the lung cyst in 59 (14.4%). Intraoperative complications were recorded in three patients (0.7%) (Fig. 2.5).

Among 78 patients, 91 early postoperative complications were identified in the present series including pneumothorax in 19 patients, pneumonia in 15, respiratory distress in 11, pleural effusion in 8, a persisting cystic lesion in 7, thoracic deformity in 7, central nervous system complications in 5, and others in 20. Of these, 11

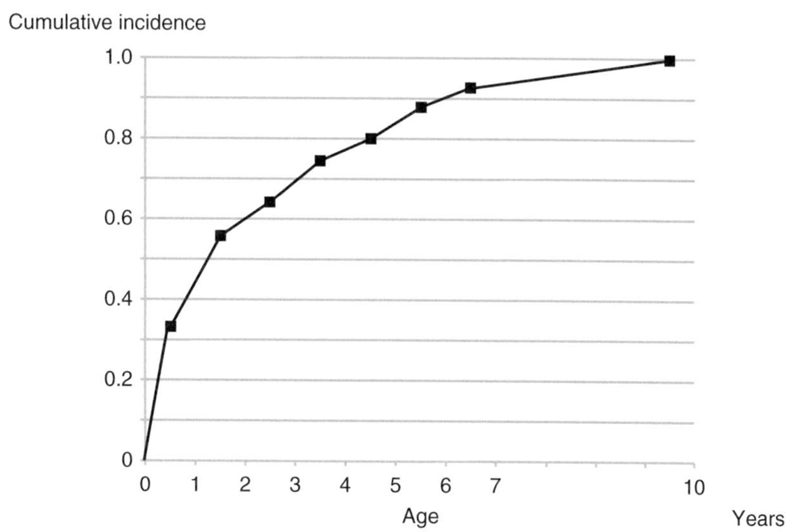


**Fig. 2.4** Cumulative incidence of CCLD symptoms. The cumulated incidence of the symptoms related to CCLD drastically increased before the age of 2 years and became 74.3% at the age of 3 years. Only 7.1% of the patients developed symptoms after the age of 6 years

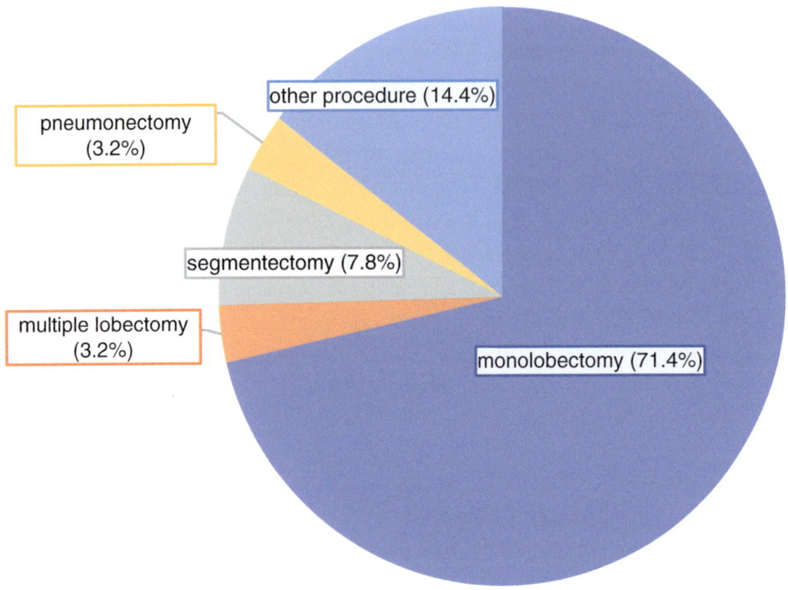


**Fig. 2.5** Types of surgery for CCLD. The types of surgery for CCLD was 292 patients (71.4%) had monolobectomy, 13 patients (3.2%) had multiple lobectomy, 32 patients (7.8%) had segmentectomy, 13 patients (3.2%) had pneumonectomy, and other procedures such as wedge resection and fenestration of the lung cyst was performed in 59 (14.4%)

patients did not have their complications improved. During the late postoperative period of more than 5 years after surgery, 40 complications were additionally identified including thoracic deformity in 30 patients, persisting lung cyst in 4 patients, and others in 6 patients. However, none of the patients in the present series have developed pulmonary cancer.

In the present series, 14 patients died most commonly during the neonatal and early infantile period. The causes of death included pulmonary hypoplasia because of CCLD in nine patients, and uncontrollable pneumothorax, expanding CCLD lesion, pulmonary hypertension, massive intracranial hemorrhage, and accompanying major anomalies in five patients, respectively.

## 2.4 Respiratory Function Measured During Late Postoperative Period

Data on the postoperative respiratory function beyond the age of 6 years was available for 22 patients. The percentage VC showed a gradual increase with age after the age of 7 years and finally reached around 90%. Interestingly, a few prenatally diagnosed patients showed definitely higher %VC values even before the age of 7 years. The averaged final %VC was significantly higher in the prenatally diagnosed patients than in the postnatally diagnosed patients (98.3 ± 11.9% vs. 81.7 ± 9.7%, $P < 0.0222$) (Fig. 2.6). However, FEV1/FVC showed no significant difference between the two patients (87.3 ± 13.7 in prenatally diagnosed cohort vs. 84.2 ± 8.3 in postnatally diagnosed cohort, $P > 0.34$).

## 2.5 Lung Lesions and Pathological Diagnosis

As shown in Table 2.3, The pathological diagnosis of resected lung specimens made by institutional pathologists included CCAM or CPAM in 247 patients, intralobar bronchopulmonary sequestration in 63 patients, extralobar bronchopulmonary sequestration in 39 patients, bronchial atresia in 66 patients, bronchogenic cyst in 15 patients, lobar emphysema in 9 patients, Bulla/Breb in 2 patients, and other diagnoses in 21 patients. Bronchial obstruction and abnormalities of the pulmonary artery were described in 23.4 and 9.5% of them, respectively.

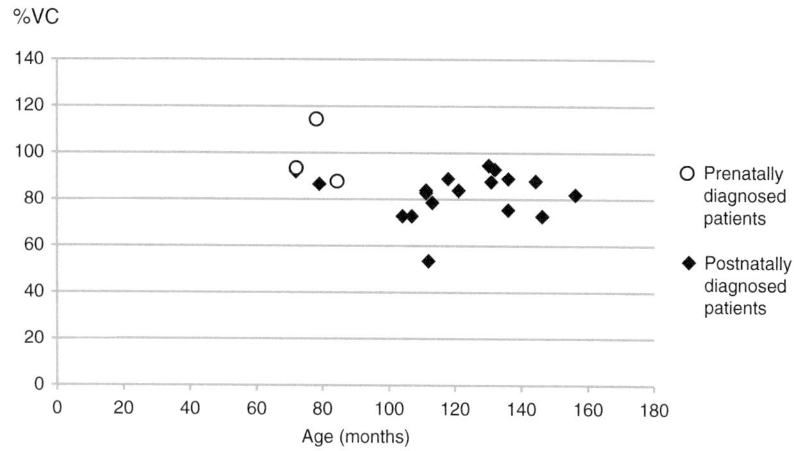


**Fig. 2.6** Postoperative %VC after grown-up. Averaged %VC at the age over 6 years was significantly higher in the prenatally diagnosed patients compared to the postnatally diagnosed patients (98.3 ± 11.9% vs. 81.7 ± 9.7%, $p < 0.0222$)

**Table 2.3** Pathological diagnosis

| Pathological diagnosis (some of them are overlapped) | $n = 428$ |
|---|---|
| CPAM | 247 |
| Intralobar bronchopulmonary sequestration | 63 |
| Extralobar bronchopulmonary sequestration | 39 |
| Bronchial atresia | 66 |
| Bronchogenic cyst | 15 |
| Lobar emphysema | 9 |
| Bulla/Breb | 2 |
| Other diagnoses | 21 |

## 2.6 Discussion

To obtain an overview of congenital cystic lung diseases (CCLD) in Japan and identify the features of prenatally and postnatally diagnosed cases, we conducted a multicenter study involving facilities with high volumes of CCLD patients.

In this study, 45.3% of cases were diagnosed prenatally. Diagnostic imaging in the fetal period was performed using ultrasonography and fetal MRI. Lesion sites were initially detected by fetal ultrasonographic examination at 12-42 weeks of gestation (median: 24 weeks), and abnormalities such as pulmonary space-occupying lesions (89.2%), mediastinal shift (51.9%), and polyhydramnios (14.0%) were identified. Furthermore, fetal hydropic changes, which have serious implications for prognosis and postnatal respiratory status, were observed in 13.6% of cases. The present study found higher rates of fetal hydrops than those reported in previous studies [1–3]. Fetal therapy was implemented for fetuses with risks like hydrops fetalis, including therapies such as steroid administration (8.1%), cyst aspiration (10.4%), and thoracoamniotic shunting (9.0%); these rates are also slightly higher than those reported previously [1–3].

Fetal lung lesion volume ratio (LVR), a ratio of lung lesion volume to head circumference, was measured at least twice during the gestational period: once at initial diagnosis and again in the third trimester. Typically, LVR tended to decrease in the third trimester. However, patients who exhibited respiratory symptoms immediately after birth had a significantly higher initial LVR measurement than the asymptomatic group. These results and those of previous studies including our own reconfirm LVR as a possible predictive risk factor [4–7]. In particular, a lack of third trimester reduction in LVR appeared to be strongly associated with postnatal respiratory distress. In addition, patients with fetal hydrops had a significantly higher LVR than patients without hydrops, both in early pregnancy and in the third trimester. These results agree with previous reports that LVR could be a predictive factor for fetal hydrops and postnatal respiratory status [1, 3, 8–11]. LVR appears to be a factor by which postnatal respiratory status could be more accurately predicted than by other imaging findings.

Although lesion reduction (LVR reduction) is seen among various CCLD in both CPAM and non-CPAM lesions [12–14], in CPAM, it is reported to be strongly associated with high risk of perinatal respiratory insufficiency [2, 6, 12, 13, 15]. In this study, however, we did not obtain results indicating a statistically significant difference in lesion reduction between CPAM patients and CCLD patients without CPAM. The main reasons for this seem to be that pathological classification of CCLD is still unclear and that many non-CPAM cases (like bronchial occlusion) exist even among those diagnosed as CPAM. In the future, it will be important to evaluate risk factors based on more accurate pathological diagnosis of CPAM.

Immediately after birth, chest retractions and tachypnea were observed in 29.8% and 29.2% of patients, respectively. Approximately 15% of neonatal patients had an APGAR score below 8. At postnatal day 30, approximately 15% of neonatal patients required respiratory support. 3.3% of patients had died. Approximately 5–10% of prenatally diagnosed patients suffered severe postnatal respiratory insufficiency and required emergency surgical intervention and intensive respiratory support in the neonatal period [2, 16].

In this study, patients who were asymptomatic at birth, developed infections of pulmonary cystic lesions at an earlier stage than that stated in previous reports. It has traditionally been thought that infectious symptoms develop after the first year of life in CPAM and at age 3–4 or later in other CCLD [14, 17]. However, in this study, one-third of patients developed symptoms of infection in the first year of life. In addition, approximately 65% of patients had symptoms of some kind by 3 years of age, and the cumulative incidence of symptoms was extremely high at 74.3% [2, 16]. We consider these results highly significant as they shed light on the natural history of CCLD from the fetal period.

Although we were able to assess later pulmonary function only in a few cases, the postoperative data obtained provides extremely valuable information. In this study, the majority of patients underwent lobectomy, and their average postoperative %VC exceeded 90% (incredibly high compared to adults after thoracic surgery) and beyond the age of 7, when lung development is considered virtually complete. Furthermore, prenatally diagnosed cases showed a significantly higher %VC at an early stage than did postnatally diagnosed cases [2, 16]. These results suggest that by receiving a prenatal diagnosis and undergoing surgery before the onset of pulmonary infection, patients may have the potential to achieve better development of the remaining lung. The results further suggest that early surgery before age 1–2 is essential even for asymptomatic patients.

Among late postoperative complications, persistent pulmonary cysts were most typically observed. The preservation of unaffected lobes appears in such cases to be the rational option for avoiding pneumonectomy and post-pneumonectomy syndrome. Depending on the patient, residual cysts are unavoidable in some cases, and these may require resection in a repeat surgery.

Despite reports that alveolar cell carcinoma develops from CPAM especially [17–19], this carcinoma, which has been thought to arise from CCLD, did not develop from CCLD in any patients during the present study [2, 16]. The incidence of carcinogenesis from cystic lung disease seems to be extremely low, but evaluation by future research is required.

## References


1. Ruchonnet-Metrailler I, Leroy-Terquem E, Stirnemann J, Cros P, Ducoin H, Hadchouel A, et al. Neonatal outcomes of prenatally diagnosed congenital pulmonary malformations. Pediatrics. 2014;133(5):e1285–91.
2. Kuroda T, Nishijima E, Maeda K, Fuchimoto Y, Hirobe S, Tazuke Y, et al. Perinatal features of congenital cystic lung diseases: results of a nationwide multicentric study in Japan. Pediatr Surg Int. 2016;32(9):827–31.
3. Kunisaki SM, Saito JM, Fallat ME, St Peter SD, Lal DR, Johnson KN, et al. Development of a multi-institutional registry for children with operative congenital lung malformations. J Pediatr Surg. 2019;S0022-3468(19):30112–5.

4. Crombleholme TM, Coleman B, Hedrick H, Liechty K, Howell L, Flake AW, et al. Cystic adenomatoid malformation volume ratio predicts outcome in prenatally diagnosed cystic adenomatoid malformation of the lung. J Pediatr Surg. 2002;37(3):331–8.
5. Aziz D, Langer JC, Tuuha SE, Ryan G, Ein SH, Kim PC. Perinatally diagnosed asymptomatic congenital cystic adenomatoid malformation: to resect or not? J Pediatr Surg. 2004;39(3):329–34. Discussion-34
6. Kuroda T, Morikawa N, Kitano Y, Sago H, Hayashi S, Honna T, et al. Clinicopathologic assessment of prenatally diagnosed lung diseases. J Pediatr Surg. 2006;41(12):2028–31.
7. Davenport M, Warne SA, Cacciaguerra S, Patel S, Greenough A, Nicolaides K. Current outcome of antenally diagnosed cystic lung disease. J Pediatr Surg. 2004;39(4):549–56.
8. Ehrenberg-Buchner S, Stapf AM, Berman DR, Drongowski RA, Mychaliska GB, Treadwell MC, et al. Fetal lung lesions: can we start to breathe easier? Am J Obstet Gynecol. 2013;208(2):151. e1–7
9. Yong PJ, Von Dadelszen P, Carpara D, Lim K, Kent N, Tessier F, et al. Prediction of pediatric outcome after prenatal diagnosis and expectant antenatal management of congenital cystic adenomatoid malformation. Fetal Diagn Ther. 2012;31(2):94–102.
10. Hellmund A, Berg C, Geipel A, Bludau M, Heydweiller A, Bachour H, et al. Prenatal diagnosis and evaluation of Sonographic predictors for intervention and adverse outcome in congenital pulmonary airway malformation. PLoS One. 2016;11(3):e0150474.
11. Girsen AI, Hintz SR, Sammour R, Naqvi A, El-Sayed YY, Sherwin K, et al. Prediction of neonatal respiratory distress in pregnancies complicated by fetal lung masses. Prenat Diagn. 2017;37(3):266–72.
12. Winters WD, Effmann EL, Nghiem HV, Nyberg DA. Disappearing fetal lung masses: importance of postnatal imaging studies. Pediatr Radiol. 1997;27(6):535–9.
13. Barret J, Chitayat D, Sermer M, Amankwah K, Morrow R, Toi A, et al. The prognostic factors in the prenatal diagnosis of the echogenic fetal lung. Prenat Diagn. 1995;15(9):849–53.
14. van Leeuwen K, Teitelbaum DH, Hirschl RB, Austin E, Adelman SH, Polley TZ, et al. Prenatal diagnosis of congenital cystic adenomatoid malformation and its postnatal presentation, surgical indications, and natural history. J Pediatr Surg. 1999;34(5):794–8. Discussion 8–9
15. Watanabe T, Ohno M, Tahara K, Tomonaga K, Fuchimoto Y, Fujino A, et al. An investigation on clinical differences between congenital pulmonary airway malformation and bronchial atresia. J Pediatr Surg. 2018;53(12):2390–3.
16. Kuroda T, Nishijima E, Maeda K, Fuchimoto Y, Hirobe S, Tazuke Y, et al. Clinical features of congenital cystic lung diseases: a report on a Nationwide multicenter study in Japan. Eur J Pediatr Surg. 2016;26(1):91–5.
17. Granata C, Gambini C, Balducci T, Toma P, Michelazzi A, Conte M, et al. Bronchioloalveolar carcinoma arising in congenital cystic adenomatoid malformation in a child: a case report and review on malignancies originating in congenital cystic adenomatoid malformation. Pediatr Pulmonol. 1998;25(1):62–6.
18. MacSweeney F, Papagiannopoulos K, Goldstraw P, Sheppard MN, Corrin B, Nicholson AG. An assessment of the expanded classification of congenital cystic adenomatoid malformations and their relationship to malignant transformation. Am J Surg Pathol. 2003;27(8):1139–46.
19. Ramos SG, Barbosa GH, Tavora FR, Jeudy J, Torres LA, Tone LG, et al. Bronchioloalveolar carcinoma arising in a congenital pulmonary airway malformation in a child: case report with an update of this association. J Pediatr Surg. 2007;42(5):E1–4.

# 3 Fetal Diagnosis and Therapy for Congenital Cystic Lung Disease

Haruhiko Sago

**Abstract**

A routine ultrasound examination during a pregnancy checkup can lead to the detection of congenital abnormalities in the fetal thorax. Congenital lung cystic disease (CLCD) is characterized by cyst formation or increased echogenicity in the fetal lung and includes congenital pulmonary airway malformation (CPAM), bronchopulmonary sequestration (BPS), bronchial atresia (BA) and, less commonly, bronchogenic cyst. The prognosis of fetuses with CLCD depends mainly on the size of the lesion and characteristics such as hydrops fetalis. The prenatal diagnosis of CLCD is made based on the following factors: the origin of blood supply, with a systemic artery supply indicating BPS; the appearance of the lung cyst, with a macrocystic type (cyst diameter ≥ 0.5 cm) suggesting CPAM and a microcystic type (cyst diameter < 0.5 cm) BA or CPAM; the lesion size, with a CPAM volume ratio > 1.6 likely to develop hydrops; the presence of hydrops fetalis and changes in the appearance, as hydrops is an ominous sign; and a reduced size or echogenicity of the lesion, which are favorable signs. The perinatal outcomes of fetuses with CLCD range from spontaneous regression to perinatal death with hydrops fetalis. The lesions in cases of CLCD seem to reach their maximal size by 28 weeks' gestation. Most cases show a favorable outcome; however, a few cases with large lesion associated with hydrops require fetal intervention for treatment. Thoraco-amniotic shunting and maternal steroid therapy are acceptable fetal treatment options for fetal CLCD in most fetal treatment centers.

**Keywords**

Bronchial atresia · Bronchopulmonary sequestration · Congenital pulmonary airway malformation · Fetal therapy · Maternal betamethasone · Thoraco-amniotic shunting

## 3.1 Introduction

With the frequent performance of routine ultrasound examinations during pregnancy checkups, various kinds of fetal congenital abnormalities have been detected in utero. Congenital lung cystic disease (CLCD) is one such example, characterized by cyst formation or increased echogenicity in the chest of the fetus. CLCD includes congenital pulmonary airway malformation (CPAM),

H. Sago (✉)
Center for Maternal-Fetal, Neonatal and Reproductive Medicine, National Center for Child Health and Development, Tokyo, Japan
e-mail: sagou-h@ncchd.go.jp


H. Sago et al. (eds.), *Congenital Cystic Lung Disease*, https://doi.org/10.1007/978-981-15-5175-8_3

formerly called congenital cystic adenomatoid malformation (CCAM), bronchopulmonary sequestration (BPS), bronchial atresia (BA) and, less commonly, bronchogenic cyst. The perinatal outcomes of fetuses with CLCD range from spontaneous regression to perinatal death with hydrops fetalis [1, 2]. Some fetuses with CLCD require fetal intervention or surgery just after birth [3, 4]. The prenatal diagnosis is therefore crucial for the perinatal management of fetuses with CLCD. Fetal therapy is an important treatment option for some fetuses with CLCD.

This chapter describes the fetal diagnosis of CLCD by ultrasound and the role of fetal therapy for CLCD.

## 3.2 Prenatal Diagnosis of CLCD

It is not difficult to detect lesions in cases of CLCD, but it is difficult to differentiate the diagnosis of CLCD. The classification of CLCD is based on the pathological findings of the lesion, considering the primary formation during the pulmonary development [5]. The new classification is based on the pulmonary development, which indicates how the lesion is primarily formed, and this classification was originally presented by Dr. Kuroda's group, as described in Chap. 1. The classification is as follows: (1) pulmonary airway malformation such as CPAM, (2) lung bud malformation such as BPS, (3) foregut malformation such as bronchogenic cyst, (4) BA, and (5) others. The prenatal diagnosis of CLCD by ultrasound imaging or magnetic resonance imaging (MRI) is thus limited.

The purpose of a prenatal diagnosis is to determine the prognosis of the fetus and develop an adequate perinatal management plan. The prognoses of fetuses with CLCD are thought to be mainly related to the characteristics and size of the lesion [3]. CPAM, BPS, and BA are the common diseases of fetal CLCD.

We herein describe the flow of the prenatal diagnosis of CLCD based on the origin of the blood supply, appearance of the lung cyst, lesion size, presence of hydrops fetalis, and changes in appearance (Fig. 3.1).

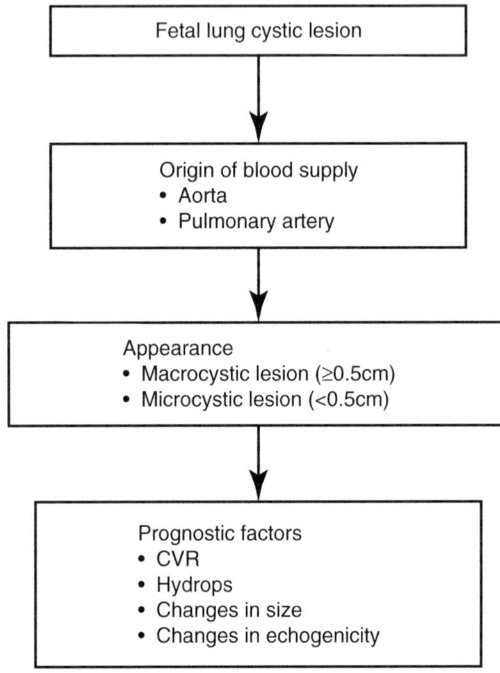


**Fig. 3.1** The flow of the prenatal diagnosis of fetal CLCD

### 3.2.1 Origin of the Blood Supply

The first step is to evaluate the origin of the blood supply of the lung lesion. Most CLCD lesions are fed by pulmonary circulation. However, BPS, which is classified as lung bud malformation, is fed by the systemic circulation. BPS is a non-functioning lung tissue mass with no communications with the bronchial tree, seen as a solid, high-echogenic lung mass with systemic feeding vessels [6]. The prenatal diagnosis of BPS involves demonstrating a systemic blood supply to the CLCD by color Doppler ultrasound (Fig. 3.2). The anomalous vessels are commonly derived from the descending aorta just below the diaphragm. There are two types of BPS manifestations: intralobar (covered by the pleura, like the normal lung) and extralobar (covered by the pleura, separate from the normal lung). These manifestations are usually difficult to distinguish by prenatal ultrasound.

Extralobar BPS is characterized by the presence of systemic artery supply and systemic venous drainage, while intralobar BPS is characterized by the presence of a systemic artery sup-

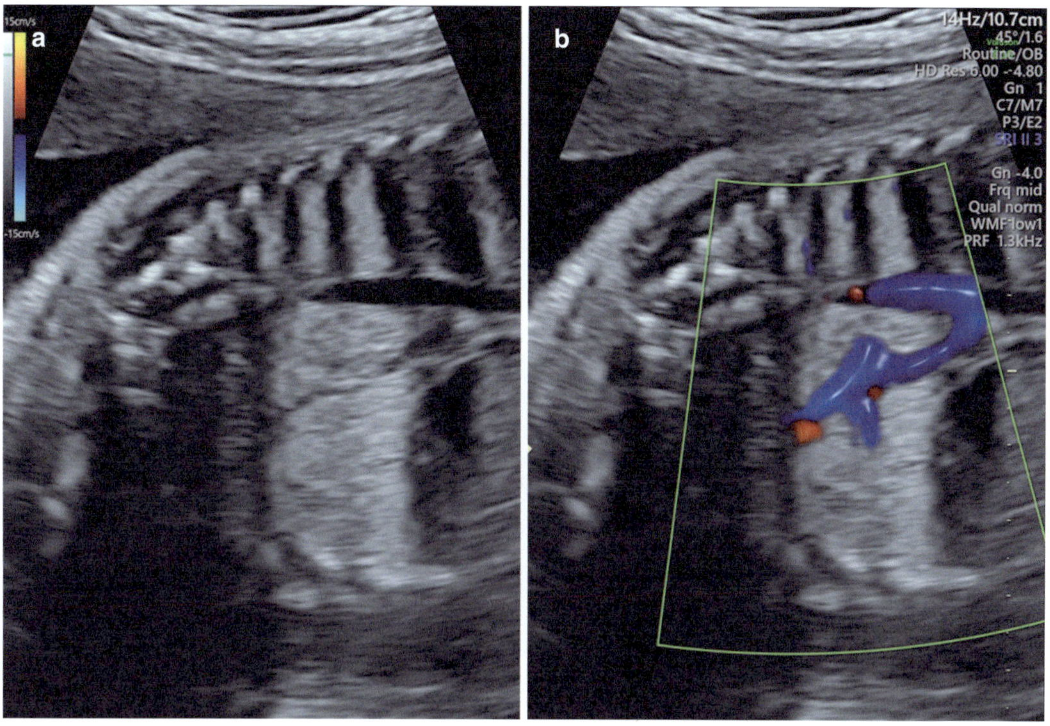


**Fig. 3.2** Ultrasound images of BPS. Without Color Doppler (**a**) and with Color Doppler (**b**). The feeding artery was derived from the aorta

ply and pulmonary venous drainage [7]. Extralobar BPS is more common than intralobar BPS in fetuses. The prognosis of BPS is usually favorable, and roughly three-quarters of prenatally diagnosed cases resolve spontaneously [1].

### 3.2.2 Appearance of the Lung Cyst

If there is no systemic blood supply, the second step is to evaluate the appearance of the CLCD lesion. Most such lesions are CPAM or BA with communication with the bronchial tree. The appearance ranges from homogeneous without a typical cyst to a multiple-cystic appearance. Stocker's classification for pathological findings uses three categories for the cyst size, as follows: >1 cm, 0.5–1 cm and < 0.5 cm [5]. Adzick et al. classified lesions into two categories based on the gross appearance on ultrasound [8]. Macrocystic lesions include single or multiple cysts ≥0.5 cm in diameter (Fig. 3.3a), whereas microcystic lesions are solid or dense cysts <0.5 cm in diameter (Fig. 3.3b). Macrocystic lesions are more likely to be CPAM, whereas microcystic lesions are likely to be BA or CPAM. However, there are some microcystic types of CPAM that show a poor prognosis [9].

### 3.2.3 Lung Cystic Lesion Size

The size rather than the type of lung cystic lesion is thought to determine the prognosis of CCLD [3]. Crombleholme et al. proposed the CCAM volume ratio (CVR), which was later termed the CPAM volume ratio (CVR), as a prognostic factor [10]. The CPAM volume is calculated using the formula for the volume of an ellipsoid (height × width × length × 0.52 [$cm^3$]) by measuring the greatest length, width, and height of the lesion (Fig. 3.4). The CVR is calculated by dividing the CPAM volume by the head circumference (cm) to adjust for any differences in the gestational age. Roughly 80% of fetuses with lung cystic lesions with a CVR

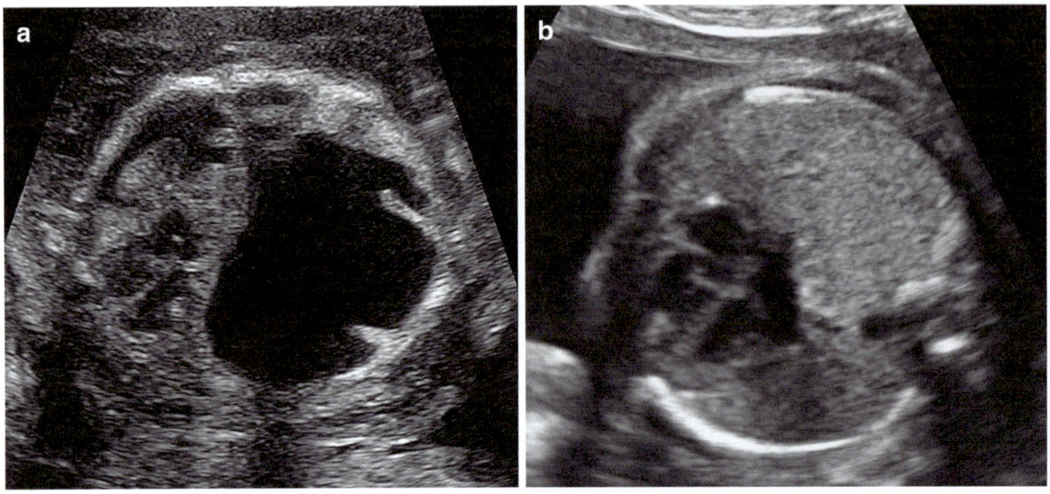


**Fig. 3.3** Ultrasound images of CLCD. Macrocystic lesion (**a**) and microcystic lesion (**b**)

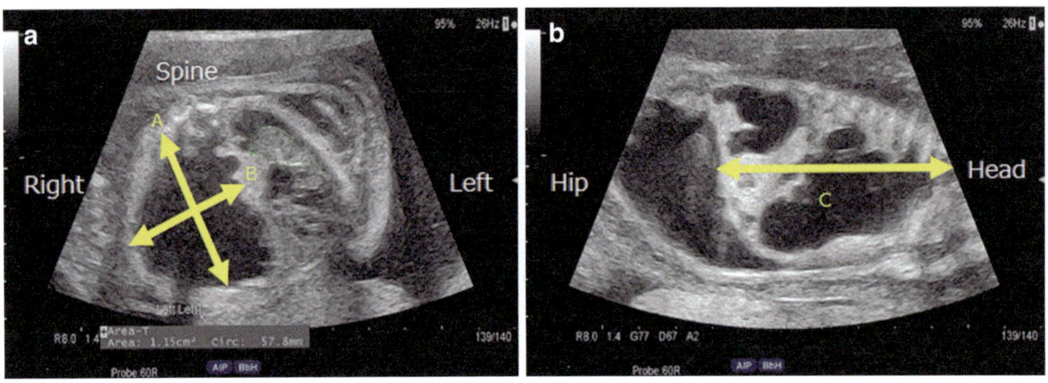


**Fig. 3.4** Measuring the CVR in the transverse section (**a**) and sagittal section (**b**). The CPAM volume is calculated as the height (A) × width (B) × length (C) × 0.52 (cm$^3$)

>1.6 develop hydrops, making a CVR >1.6 a useful size predictor for the development of hydrops [10]. A maximum CVR >1.0 is also a size predictor for respiratory morbidity requiring surgical resection after birth [11].

### 3.2.4 Presence of Hydrops and Changes in the Appearance

The most ominous sign of CCLD is hydrops fetalis. Hydrops is the result of the compression of vena cava and heart by a large lung mass. Adzick et al. described 134 cases of prenatally diagnosed CPAM, the large series of prenatal cases [1]. Of the 25 cases of large CPAM with hydrops that were followed expectantly, all fetuses died in utero or after birth. Therefore, the presence of hydrops constitutes an indication for fetal intervention. Another useful bit of information for predicting the prognosis is the change in the size and appearance over time; more specifically, a reduction in the size or echogenicity of the lesion is a favorable sign [12]. CPAM lesions are thought to reach their maximal size by 28 weeks' gestation [3]. BA usually shows reduced echogenicity in the third trimester.

## 3.3 Fetal Therapy

Fetal intervention is considered a treatment option for fetuses with life-threatening CCLD [1, 4, 13]. Fetuses with large CCLD and hydrops are at a high risk for fetal or neonatal death. The usefulness of fetal therapy is assessed by balancing the favorable effects and invasiveness to the mother and fetus. Various therapies, such as thoraco-amniotic shunting (TAS), fetal surgical resection, maternal steroid therapy, and laser therapy, have been attempted; however, only retrospective case studies are available at present [4]. TAS and maternal steroid therapy are considered acceptable options for fetal intervention in most fetal treatment centers.

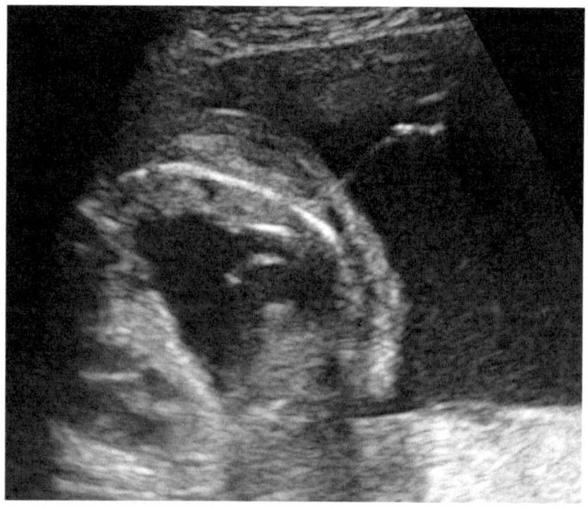

**Fig. 3.5** Ultrasound image after thoraco-amniotic shunt insertion to the cyst

### 3.3.1 TAS

TAS is commonly used for fetuses with primary hydrothorax accompanying hydrops to drain the pleural effusion. BPS is known to be associated with pleural effusion, and the development of hydrops in BPS fetuses with pleural effusion leads to perinatal death. Therefore, TAS following thoracocentesis is performed for fetal cases of hydrothorax and hydrops associated with BPS.

We previously reported three cases of fetuses with BPS associated with pleural effusion and hydrops that were successfully treated by TAS [14]. A "double-basket catheter" (Hakko Co., Nagano, Japan) is used for TAS in Japan. It was developed in Japan in the 1990s initially for vesico-amniotic shunting. Riley et al. reported the outcomes of 103 fetuses with BPS [7]. Eight (8%) developed hydrothorax, and four (4%) developed hydrops. Only three (3%) fetuses underwent TAS with subsequent resolution of hydrops. BPSs have a tendency to shrink after 28 weeks' gestation; however, a few cases still require fetal treatment.

TAS is also applied for fetuses with macrocystic CPAM containing a large predominant cyst to drain the cyst fluid (Fig. 3.5) [15]. TAS is considered in cases with a large cyst with marked mediastinal shift and/or hydrops and a CVR > 1.6 [16]. Thoracocentesis can be used to assess the degree of shrinkage of the cyst. However, the reaccumulation of fluid in the cyst necessitates TAS. A literature search found 98 fetuses with macrocystic CPAM who had been treated by TAS [16]. The survival rates for fetuses with and without hydrops were 77% (53/69) and 90% (37/41), respectively. Therefore, TAS for macrocystic CPAM with a large predominant cyst is an acceptable treatment option. Obstruction and displacement of the catheter are major complications associated with TAS.

### 3.3.2 Fetal Surgical Resection

Microcystic CPAM cannot be treated by TAS. Surgical resection by open fetal surgery is an available treatment option in utero. Open fetal surgical resection of CPAM has been attempted at a few fetal treatment centers in the United States. Adzick et al. reported the largest series of 24 cases of CPAM with fetal surgical resection between 21 and 31 weeks of gestation [17]. Thirteen (54%) fetuses survived, and 11 (46%) died. Seven of the 11 non-survivors died during the operation. Cass et al. reported three CPAM cases with fetal surgical resection [18]. One of the three fetuses died during open fetal surgery. We experienced one case of open fetal surgery for microcytic CPAM with hydrops [9]. The operation was successfully performed at 28 weeks' gestation. However, emergent Caesarean section was performed the next day due to prolonged bradycardia of the fetus, and the neonate ultimately died shortly after birth. The overall survival of fetal lobectomy in three centers in the United States was 52% (28/54) [13, 17, 18]. The risk with open fetal surgical resection for the fetus is extremely high, and this approach additionally carries perinatal and maternal risks, such as preterm premature rupture of the membrane, preterm labor, pulmonary edema, transfusion and uterine rupture. Fetal surgical resection of CPAM is not acceptable in most fetal treatment centers.

### 3.3.3 Maternal Steroid Therapy

There is no reliable treatment option for huge microcystic CPAM. Tsao et al. reported three fetuses with large CPAM and hydrops that showed unexpected resolution after maternal betamethasone injection to promote maturation of the fetal lung for preterm delivery [19]. The standard regimen for steroid therapy is injection of 12 mg of betamethasone twice to the mother, 24 hours apart. Peranteau et al. reported 11 cases of CPAM with maternal betamethasone administration [20]. The survival rate was 100%. Resolution of hydrops was seen in 80% (4/5) of cases, and a decrease in the CVR was seen in 73% of cases. Morris et al. reported 15 CPAM cases of betamethasone therapy, with 54% showing the resolution of hydrops and a 53% survival rate [21]. Curran et al. reported 13 cases of steroid therapy with 78% showing the resolution of hydrops and an 85% survival rate [22]. The response of CPAM to maternal betamethasone administration reportedly varies. Spontaneous resolution of hydrops in CPAM has also been observed [23]. More evidence is needed in order to establish maternal steroid therapy as a reliable treatment option. The underlying pathophysiology is speculated to involve the effects of steroids on augmenting the maturation of the lung lesion. Maternal betamethasone therapy is acceptable for fetuses with large microcystic CPAM with hydrops for which there is no other viable therapy, as no surgical procedure is required.

### 3.3.4 Other Fetal Therapies

Attempts at ultrasound-guided laser therapy for CCAM have been reported [24]. The laser fiber is inserted into the lung lesion via an 18-G needle. The CPAM is photocoagulated using an Nd:YAG laser. Only a few reports of such cases are available. There are some reports of laser therapy for fetuses with BPS [25], with the feeding vessels targeted for laser photocoagulation. Sclerotherapy under ultrasound guidance has also been attempted to treat fetal CPAM and BPS [26, 27]. A sclerosing agent is percutaneously inserted into the CPAM. Fourteen cases of CPAM and four cases of BPS have been reported to date [27]. We believe that laser therapy or sclerotherapy is not warranted at present due to the lack of substantial supporting evidence.

## References


1. Adzick NS, Harrison MR, Crombleholme TM, Flake AW, Howell LJ. Fetal lung lesions: management and outcome. Am J Obstet Gynecol. 1998;179(4):884–9.
2. Laberge JM, Flageole H, Pugash D, Khalife S, Blair G, Filiatrault D, Russo P, Lees G, Wilson RD. Outcome of the prenatally diagnosed congenital cystic adenomatoid lung malformation: a Canadian experience. Fetal Diagn Ther. 2001;16(3):178–86.
3. Adzick NS. Management of fetal lung lesions. Clin Perinatol. 2009;36(2):363–76.
4. Witlox RS, Lopriore E, Oepkes D. Prenatal interventions for fetal lung lesions. Prenat Diagn. 2011;31(7):628–36.
5. Stocker JT, Madewell JE, Drake RM. Congenital cystic adenomatoid malformation of the lung. Classification and morphologic spectrum. Hum Pathol. 1977;8(2):155–71.
6. Hernanz-Schulman M, Stein SM, Neblett WW, Atkinson JB, Kirchner SG, Heller RM, Merrill WH, Fleischer AC. Pulmonary sequestration: diagnosis with color Doppler sonography and a new theory of associated hydrothorax. Radiology. 1991;180(3):817–21.
7. Riley JS, Urwin JW, Oliver ER, Coleman BG, Khalek N, Moldenhauer JS, Spinner SS, Hedrick HL, Adzick NS, Peranteau WH. Prenatal growth characteristics and pre/postnatal management of bronchopulmonary sequestrations. J Pediatr Surg. 2018;53(2):265–9.
8. Adzick NS, Harrison MR, Glick PL, Golbus MS, Anderson RL, Mahony BS, Callen PW, Hirsch JH, Luthy DA, Filly RA, et al. Fetal cystic adenomatoid

malformation: prenatal diagnosis and natural history. J Pediatr Surg. 1985;20(5):483–8.
9. Kitano Y, Chiba T, Kuroda T, Sago H, et al. Open fetal surgery for congenital cystic adenomatoid malformation complicated with fetal hydrops – a case report. Nihon Syusanki-Shinseijishi. 2005;41(1):67–72.
10. Crombleholme TM, Coleman B, Hedrick H, Liechty K, Howell L, Flake AW, Johnson M, Adzick NS. Cystic adenomatoid malformation volume ratio predicts outcome in prenatally diagnosed cystic adenomatoid malformation of the lung. J Pediatr Surg. 2002;37(3):331–8.
11. Ehrenberg-Buchner S, Stapf AM, Berman DR, Drongowski RA, Mychaliska GB, Treadwell MC, Kunisaki SM. Fetal lung lesions: can we start to breathe easier? Am J Obstet Gynecol. 2013;208(2): 151. e1-7
12. Kunisaki SM, Ehrenberg-Buchner S, Dillman JR, Smith EA, Mychaliska GB, Treadwell MC. Vanishing fetal lung malformations: prenatal sonographic characteristics and postnatal outcomes. J Pediatr Surg. 2015;50(6):978–82.
13. Grethel EJ, Wagner AJ, Clifton MS, Cortes RA, Farmer DL, Harrison MR, Nobuhara KK, Lee H. Fetal intervention for mass lesions and hydrops improves outcome: a 15-year experience. J Pediatr Surg. 2007;42(1):117–23.
14. Hayashi S, Sago H, Kitano Y, Kuroda T, Honna T, Nakamura T, Ito Y, Kitagawa M, Natori M. Fetal pleuroamniotic shunting for bronchopulmonary sequestration with hydrops. Ultrasound Obstet Gynecol. 2006;28(7):963–7.
15. Schrey S, Kelly EN, Langer JC, Davies GA, Windrim R, Seaward PG, Ryan G. Fetal thoracoamniotic shunting for large macrocystic congenital cystic adenomatoid malformations of the lung. Ultrasound Obstet Gynecol. 2012;39(5):515–20.
16. Litwińska M, Litwińska E, Janiak K, Piaseczna-Piotrowska A, Gulczyńska E, Szaflik K. Thoracoamniotic shunts in macrocystic lung lesions: case series and review of the literature. Fetal Diagn Ther. 2017;41(3):179–83.
17. Adzick NS. Open fetal surgery for life-threatening fetal anomalies. Semin Fetal Neonatal Med. 2010;15(1):1–8.
18. Cass DL, Olutoye OO, Cassady CI, Moise KJ, Johnson A, Papanna R, Lazar DA, Ayres NA, Belleza-Bascon B. Prenatal diagnosis and outcome of fetal lung masses. J Pediatr Surg. 2011;46(2):292–8.
19. Tsao K, Hawgood S, Vu L, Hirose S, Sydorak R, Albanese CT, Farmer DL, Harrison MR, Lee H. Resolution of hydrops fetalis in congenital cystic adenomatoid malformation after prenatal steroid therapy. J Pediatr Surg. 2003;38(3):508–10.
20. Peranteau WH, Wilson RD, Liechty KW, Johnson MP, Bebbington MW, Hedrick HL, Flake AW, Adzick NS. Effect of maternal betamethasone administration on prenatal congenital cystic adenomatoid malformation growth and fetal survival. Fetal Diagn Ther. 2007;22(5):365–71.
21. Morris LM, Lim FY, Livingston JC, Polzin WJ, Crombleholme TM. High-risk fetal congenital pulmonary airway malformations have a variable response to steroids. J Pediatr Surg. 2009;44(1):60–5.
22. Curran PF, Jelin EB, Rand L, Hirose S, Feldstein VA, Goldstein RB, Lee H. Prenatal steroids for microcystic congenital cystic adenomatoid malformations. J Pediatr Surg. 2010;45(1):145–50.
23. Diamond IR, Wales PW, Smith SD, Fecteau A. Survival after CCAM associated with ascites: a report of a case and review of the literature. J Pediatr Surg. 2003;38(9):E1–3.
24. Ong SS, Chan SY, Ewer AK, Jones M, Young P, Kilby MD. Laser ablation of foetal microcystic lung lesion: successful outcome and rationale for its use. Fetal Diagn Ther. 2006;21(5):471–4.
25. Oepkes D, Devlieger R, Lopriore E, Klumper FJ. Successful ultrasound-guided laser treatment of fetal hydrops caused by pulmonary sequestration. Ultrasound Obstet Gynecol. 2007;29(4): 457–9.
26. Bermúdez C, Pérez-Wulff J, Arcadipane M, Bufalino G, Gómez L, Flores L, Sosa C, Bornick PW, Kontopoulos E, Quintero RA. Percutaneous fetal sclerotherapy for congenital cystic adenomatoid malformation of the lung. Fetal Diagn Ther. 2008;24(3):237–40.
27. Abbasi N, Morency AM, Langer JC, Chiu PPL, Chami R, Windrim R, Keunen J, Seaward G, Ryan G. Fetal Sclerotherapy for Hydropic congenital cystic Adenomatoid malformations of the lung refractory to steroids: a case report and review of the literature. Fetal Diagn Ther. 2019;21:1–10.

# 4 Fetal Diagnostic Imaging of Congenital Cystic Lung Disease

Osamu Miyazaki

**Abstract**

Cystic disease of the fetal lung covers a wide spectrum of lesions. Their etiology is unknown clearly, but it is thought to be caused by an obstruction or malformation sequence occurring in early gestation. In this chapter, we evaluated the imaging findings and pathological characterization of the fetal diagnostic imaging of congenital cystic lung disease including congenital pulmonary airway malformation (CPAM), bronchopulmonary sequestration (BPS), bronchial atresia (BA), congenital lobar emphysema (CLE), and Congenital bronchogenic cyst. These are usually evaluated in the prenatal period with fetal ultrasonography (US), but fetal magnetic resonance (MR) imaging is a well-established modality that is used as an additional technique in difficult diagnostic situations. MR imaging can provide excellent soft tissue contrast with more accurate analysis of the fetal anatomy and superior differentiation between the abnormalities.

**Keywords**

Fetus (line feed) prenatal diagnosis · Magnetic resonance imaging (MRI) · Fetal ultrasonography Congenital pulmonary airway malformation (CPAM) · Bronchopulmonary sequestration (BPS) · Single-shot turbo spin echo (SSTSE) · Balanced-steady state free precession (b-SSFP)

## 4.1 Introduction

Congenital lung abnormalities (CLAs) are heterogenous entities consisting of bronchopulmonary anomalies, vascular anomalies or a combination of these. The most common CLA is congenital pulmonary airway malformation (CPAM), followed by bronchopulmonary sequestration (BPS), bronchial atresia (BA), bronchogenic cyst and congenital lobar emphysema (CLE) or congenital lobar overinflation (CLO). These entities account for more than 95% of the CLA group [1].

Prenatal diagnosis of CLA is sometimes difficult and confusing because of the presence of complex, hybrid lesions with combined vascular and bronchopulmonary abnormalities or overlapping findings between different lesions. Some of these diseases look similar and cannot be differentiated from each other.

O. Miyazaki (✉)
Department of Radiology, National Center for Child Health and Development, Tokyo, Japan
e-mail: miyazaki-o@ncchd.go.jp



H. Sago et al. (eds.), *Congenital Cystic Lung Disease*, https://doi.org/10.1007/978-981-15-5175-8_4

Accurate prenatal diagnosis of CLA is important because there is prenatal variability in clinical evolution and outcomes, from complete involution in utero to progressive growth and secondary complications [1, 2], and the natural history and treatment of these lesions differ depending on the lesion and its type. Accurate characterization allows better prenatal counseling and appropriate postnatal management.

With advances in both fetal ultrasonography (US) and magnetic resonance imaging (MRI), CLAs and other abnormalities of the fetal thorax are increasingly being recognized antenatally [3]. Routine US including the color Doppler method has been used in daily practice for a long time to detect and follow-up CLA [4]. Most lung lesions can be detected on routine 18- to 20-week US [2]. As with advancing US technology, prenatal MRI has been increasingly used in the further evaluation of fetal lung lesions and has been shown to be particularly useful when US findings are inconclusive [2]. Alamo et al. suggested the aims of supplementary fetal MRI as follows: (1) to further characterize the morphology of the lesion and its effects on normal lung, (2) to determine the volumes of both the normal and abnormal lung, and (3) to further inform the discussion concerning intervention (termination of pregnancy, immediate delivery, thoracoamniotic shunting or puncture of a dominant cyst, or administration of prenatal corticosteroids for treatment of severe types with small cysts such as CPAM, etc. [1]). In the literature researched by Beydon et al., no clear superiority was found for fetal MRI over US in the prenatal evaluation of CLA, but US better demonstrated systemic feeding vessels and MRI cysts and normal lung adjacent to the lesion [4].

## 4.2 Safety, Magnetic Fields, and Gestational Age in Fetal MRI

According to the American College of Radiology (ACR)—Society for Pediatric Radiology (SPR) practice parameters for the safe and optimal application of fetal MRI guidelines, current data have not conclusively documented any deleterious effects of 1.5 Tesla MR imaging on the developing fetus. Therefore, no special considerations are recommended during any trimester of pregnancy [5].

Ray et al. evaluated long-term safety after exposure to MRI in the first trimester of pregnancy ($n$ = 1737), and they concluded that exposure to 1.5 Tesla MRI during the first trimester of pregnancy compared with non-exposure was not associated with increased risk of harm to the fetus or in early childhood [6]. Victoria et al. described their preliminary experience in imaging the fetus at 3 Tesla MRI, which has a signal-to-noise ratio (SNR) that is superior to 1.5 Tesla when the technique is optimized [7]. Cartier et al. reported no adverse effects with regard to neonatal hearing or fetal growth in healthy neonates who were variably exposed to 3 Tesla MRI in utero during MRI for various clinical maternal or fetal indications at any gestational age [8]. In fact, Chapman et al. reported that in their questionnaire survey conducted in 2018, the majority of radiologists (68.6%) utilize 1.5 Tesla scanning platforms, and a small percentage (6.7%) exclusively uses 3 Tesla imaging [9].

Knowledge of the gestational age of the pregnancy is important for planning the examination and positioning the surface coil. The ACR-SPR guideline recommends that "prior to 18 weeks gestational age the fetal MRI study can give limited diagnostic information due to the small size of the fetus and fetal movement. If the examination is limited by early gestational age then it may need to be repeated later" [5].

## 4.3 Fetal MR Image Acquisition Technique and Normal Lung Anatomy

A fast imaging technique is essential for fetal MRI to decrease motion artifacts, and hence single-shot turbo spin echo (SSTSE) and balanced-steady state free precession (b-SSFP) sequences are widely used [10]. The speed of b-SSFP and its high SNR have made it useful in fetal MR imaging [11]. However, an SSTSE sequence is essential for detecting aberrant arteries in the diagnosis of BPS on fetal MRI (The details will be described later). b-SSFP is thought to be safer for the fetus due to the lower radiofrequency (RF) absorption than occurs with an SSTSE sequence [11].

T2-weighted images (T2WIs) are useful for evaluating normal lung anatomy. The lungs typically contain a significant amount of alveolar fluid, which is homogeneously hyperintense relative to the chest wall muscle on T2WI. In cases where there is lung compression, the amount of alveolar fluid is decreased, resulting in a more hypointense signal [12]. Other structures—trachea, bronchi, and lungs—reveal homogeneous hyperintensity on T2WI in comparison to chest wall muscles, because they contain a significant amount of amniotic and alveolar fluid. Kuwashima et al. reported that the ratio of fetal lung-to-liver intensity ranged from 2.06–3.70 (mean 2.79) in infants without pulmonary hypoplasia within the gestational age range of 26–37 weeks [13]. T1-weighted sequences can be performed to evaluate the liver and bowel in patients with congenital diaphragmatic hernia.

## 4.4 Image Findings

### 4.4.1 Congenital Pulmonary Airway Malformation (CPAM)

CPAM, formerly known as congenital cystic adenomatoid malformation (CCAM), is a heterogeneous group of lesions caused by overgrowth of mesenchymal elements and impairment of normal alveolar development. The term CPAM has been recommended as being preferable to the term CCAM because the lesions are cystic in only three of the five types (type 1, 2, and 4) and adenomatoid in only one (type 3) [3]. Most CPAMs involve the pulmonary vascular circuit and there is normal communication with the bronchial tree. CPAM cysts are lined by respiratory ciliated epithelium.

Stocker et al. has pathologically classified CPAM into three types according to cyst size and histologic resemblance to the segments of the developing bronchial tree and air spaces as follows [14]. Type 1 macrocystic CPAM is characterized by single/multiple cysts greater than 20 mm in diameter. This accounts for approximately half of all CPAM cases in the postnatal period (Figs. 4.1, 4.2). Type 2 lesions are charac-

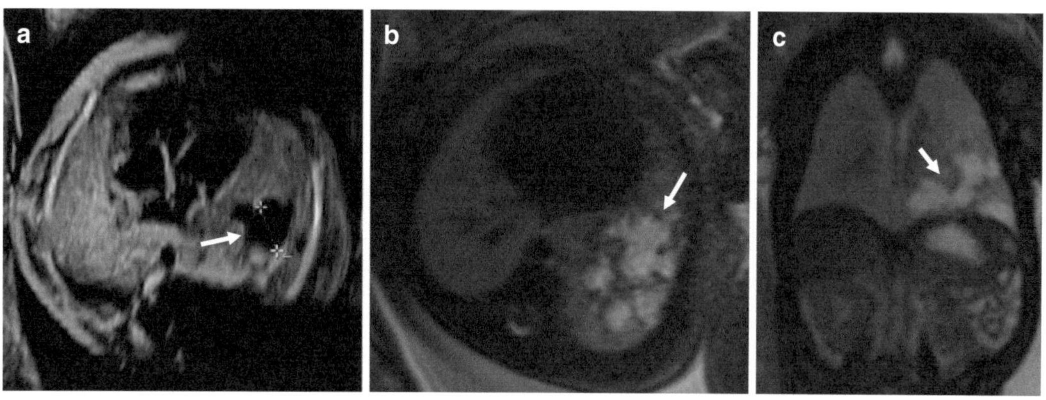


**Fig. 4.1** Congenital pulmonary airway malformation (CPAM) type 1. Fetal US at 27 gestational weeks (**a**), fetal MRI at 31 gestational weeks (axial SSTSE sequence [**b**], coronal b-SSFP sequence [**c**]), contrast-enhanced chest CT at 1 day old (**d**, **e**). Note hypoechoic area at left lower lung on fetal US (**a**, arrow) as macrocystic type. An axial SSTSE (T2WI) sequence (**b**, arrow) and coronal b-SSFP sequence (**c**, arrow) revealed multiple well-defined irregular-shaped cystic components in the left lower lobe. The surface of these cystic lesions has a bumpy appearance. These characteristic fetal images suggest typical Type 1 CPAM. Contrast-enhanced chest CT performed at 1 day old (**d**, **e**) revealed that fluid content had been replaced by air. The patient underwent surgical treatment soon after chest CT because of respiratory insufficiency. Final diagnosis of CPAM type 1 was based on pathological examination

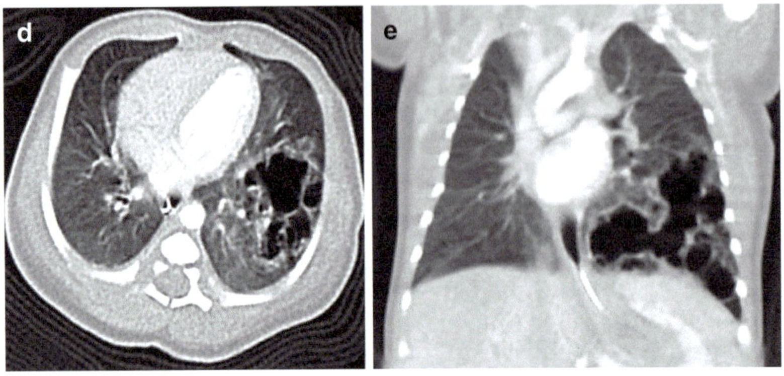

**Fig. 4.1** (continued)

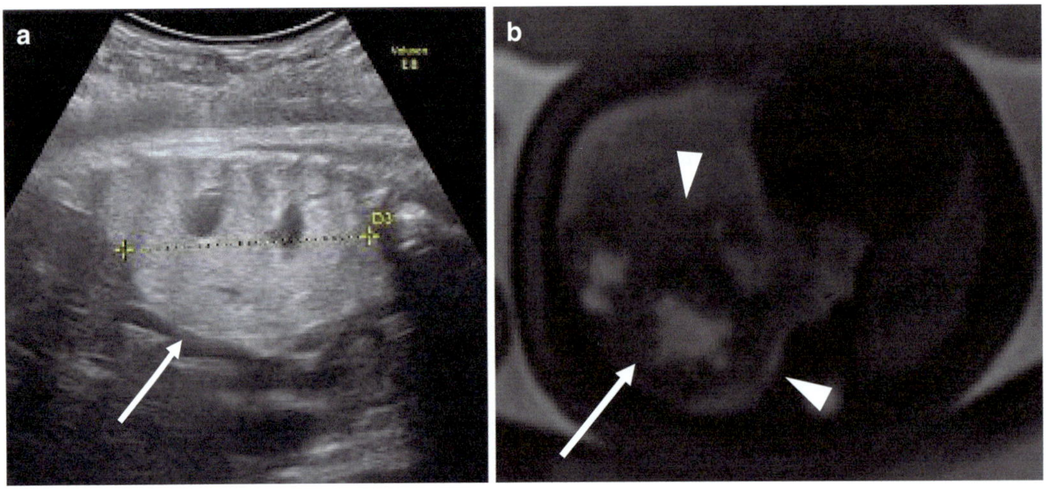

**Fig. 4.2** Rare solid and cystic type CPAM type 1 with T2-hypointense components. Fetal US at 37 gestational weeks (**a**), fetal MRI at 36 gestational weeks (axial, sagittal, coronal view of SSTSE sequence [**b**, **c**, **d**]), chest radiograph at 0 day old (**e**), axial and coronal contrast-enhanced chest CT at 1 day old (**f**, **g**). Note hyperechoic, homogeneous, expansile area in right lower lung on sagittal fetal US with several small hypoechoic areas (a, arrow). All three planes of SSTSE (T2WI) sequence (**b**, **c**, **d**) revealed multiple irregular, high-intensity areas (arrows), which correspond to the cystic cavities observed with fetal US. These areas are surrounded by a thick, low-signal-intensity component (arrowheads). Based on these findings, we considered that the diagnosis was atypical CPAM type 1, although neoplastic entities such as pleuropulmonary blastoma and rhabdomyosarcoma were also in the differential diagnosis. On plain chest radiograph (**e**), this lesion shows a large soft-tissue density in the right middle–lower lung that is partially aerated. Mediastinal content is slightly shifted toward the left side. On contrast-enhanced chest CT (**f**, **g**), this lesion is slightly enhanced in the parenchyma around the cavity. Air and fluid density can be seen in the cavity (**f**, arrow). The patient underwent surgical treatment soon after chest CT because of respiratory insufficiency. The final diagnosis of CPAM type 1 was based on pathological examination

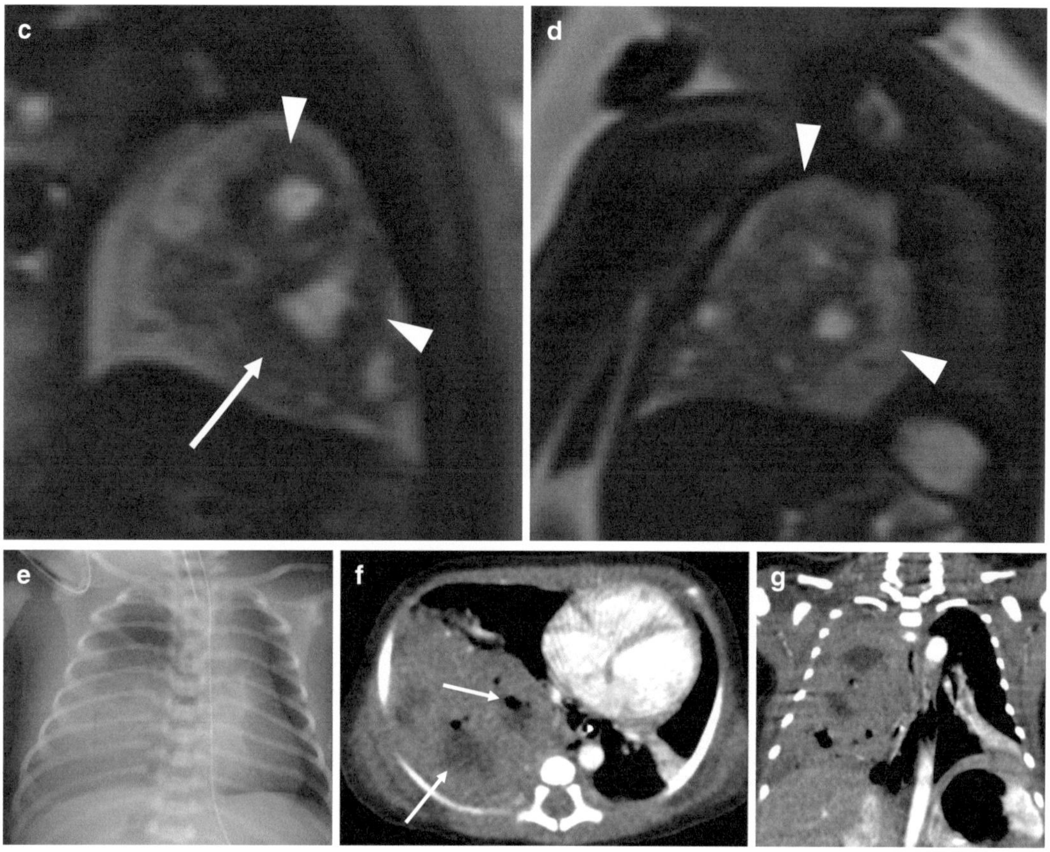


**Fig. 4.2** (continued)

terized by macroscopic cysts ranging from 5 to 20 mm in diameter (Fig. 4.3), and type 3 lesions are predominately solid with microcystic components involving almost all of the affected lung lobes (Fig. 4.4).

Recently, two additional subtypes of CPAM have been added to the classification (type 0 and type 4). CPAM type 0 is characterized by acinar dysplasia/agenesis and is very rare [14]. CPAM type 4 is composed of large thin-walled cysts, often 8–10 cm in diameter, in older infants and young children [14].

Adzick et al. suggested modified Stocker's three types and dividing CCAM into two major groups based on gross anatomy and US findings [15]. The two categories were based on the predominant component of the lesion (cystic or solid): the macrocystic group contains single or multiple cysts ≥5 mm in diameter, while the microcystic tumors are more solid and bulky, with cysts <5 mm in diameter. The variants are readily differentiated on prenatal ultrasound because the macrocystic type appears as fluid-filled lesions, whereas the microcystic lesions have innumerable interfaces that return the ultrasound beam and therefore appear solid. This simple classification into two types, either cystic or solid, has become the gold standard of in-utero CCAM/CPAM diagnosis and prognosis [16].

On prenatal US, CPAM appears as a macrocystic mass (Fig. 4.1a), microcystic solid mass (Fig. 4.4a, b), or a complex mass with both cystic and solid (echogenic) components (Figs. 4.1a, 4.2a). Solid masses are typically hyperechoic compared with normal fetal lung in the second trimester (Figs. 4.2, 4.4), and often become isoechoic with the normal lung and invisible on US in the third trimester [17].

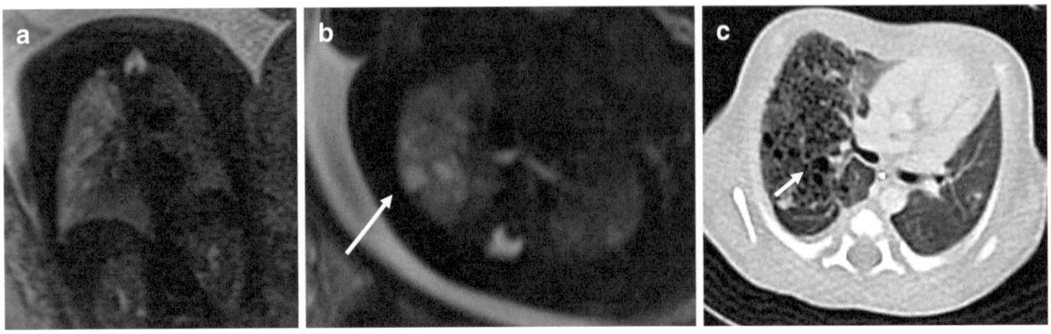

**Fig. 4.3** Congenital pulmonary airway malformation (CPAM) type 2. Fetal MRI at 33 gestational weeks (coronal [**a**], and axial [**b**], SSTSE sequence), contrast-enhanced chest CT at 0 day old (**c**). On fetal MRI, multiple small cystic areas were visualized in right upper and middle lung field. These cysts were less than 10 mm in diameter and would appear to be relatively smaller than typical CPAM type 1 lesions (**b**, arrow). CT scan soon after birth showed a complex cystic mass (**c**, arrow) in the right lung. All the cysts are small (<2 cm), a finding that is consistent with a small cyst CPAM. Pathologically, CPAM type 2 was proven without bronchial atresia

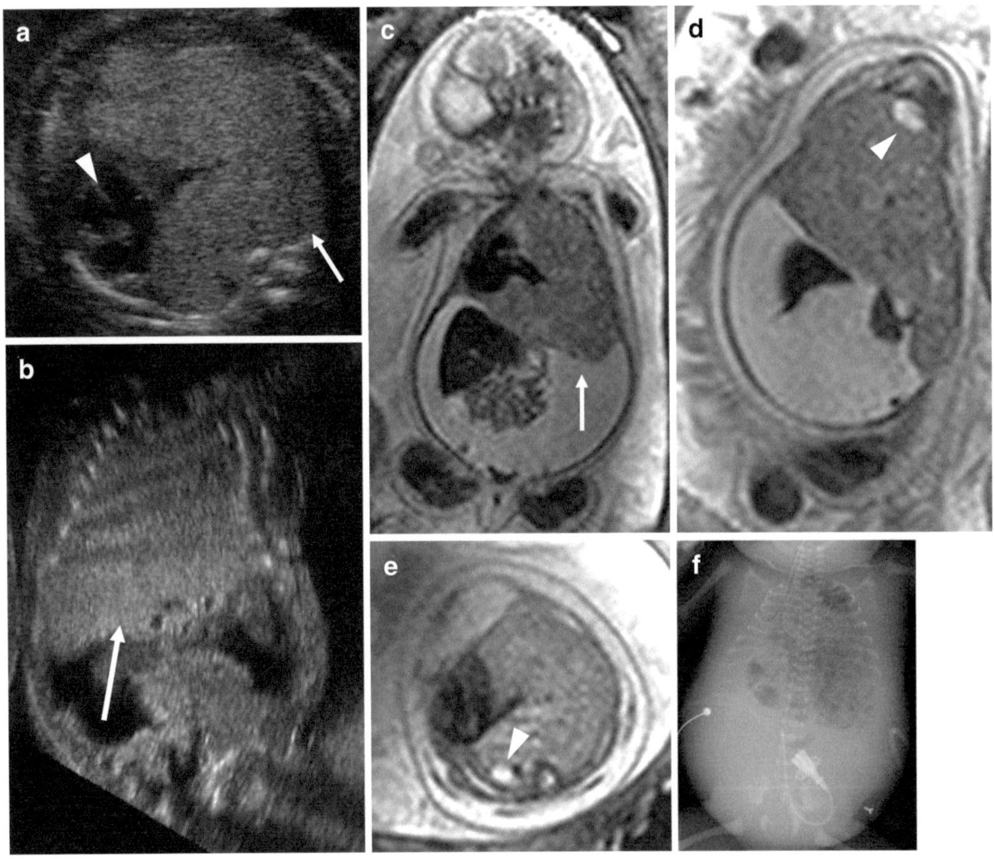

**Fig. 4.4** Congenital pulmonary airway malformation (CPAM) type 3 as solid-appearing CPAM. Fetal US (**a**, **b**) and MRI at 25 gestational weeks (coronal [**c**], and sagittal [**d**], axial [**e**] of SSTSE sequence), chest and abdominal radiograph at 0 day old (**f**). Axial and sagittal fetal US images showed a large hyperechoic lesion (**a**, **b** arrow) in the left hemithorax without any cystic lesion. Heart and mediastinum were markedly compressed by expanded lung parenchyma toward right side (**a**, arrowhead). The finding on fetal MRI was very similar that on US. However, fetal MRI demonstrated small cystic areas within the mass (**d**, **e** arrowheads). Note that the diaphragm is intact (**c**, arrow). Chest radiograph (**f**) soon after the birth showed marked distended left lung with inhomogeneous abnormal aeration. The lesion was pathologically proved to represent a CPAM type 3

Microcystic lesion appears as a solid hyperechoic mass because of the numerous acoustic interfaces created by small cysts measuring less than 5 mm in diameter (Fig. 4.4).

CPAMs are usually unilateral and unilobar with a slight preference for the lower lobes. Approximately 40% of CPAMs increase in size during pregnancy, with the most rapid growth occurring between 20 and 24 weeks' gestation, after which growth peaks and plateaus [17].

Fetal MRI is also useful in the diagnosis of CPAMs. CPAMs appear as a high signal intensity mass compared with normal lung parenchyma on T2WI, in the second trimester of pregnancy. Otherwise, during the third trimester, CPAMs may appear on T2WI to be of any intensity: high, isointense, or low-signal. Therefore, identification of a macrocystic component and/or distortion of the vascular structure is highly suggestive of CPAMs [17]. However, as mentioned above, CPAMs sometimes appear to have unusually low signal intensity on T2WI (Fig. 4.2), resembling a solid tumor/mass-like component [18, 19]. Recently, Victoria et al. reported six cases with low-signal lesions on fetal MRI using T2WI. Five of these lesions were CPAMs; one was a congenital peribronchial myofibroblastic tumor (CPMT) [19]. On pathological examination, these areas correlated with immature parenchymal development and increased mesenchymal tissue [19]. They concluded that radiologists, obstetricians, and fetal surgeons alike are aware of these lesions.

## 4.5 Bronchopulmonary Sequestration (BPS)

BPSs represent a cystic developmental malformation composed of nonfunctioning pulmonary tissue, which lacks communication with the tracheobronchial tree and is supplied by a systemic artery.

BPS is the second most common cause of a congenital lung mass (approximately 1.1–1.8% of all of cases where pulmonary resection is performed) [17]. Although BPS occurs primarily as an isolated lesion, it is known to have associated anomalies in approximately 8% of cases and to be associated with a CPAM in 25% of cases, forming a hybrid lesion [17]. BPS is preferentially located in the left lower thorax in 65–90% of cases [17].

Sequestrations are classified as intralobar sequestration (ILS, the majority of lesions are thought to be acquired), and extralobar sequestration (ELS, thought to be congenital); both can have cystic components.

ELS has its own pleura and no communication to the bronchial tree, while ILS does not have separate pleura and may communicate with the bronchial tree. ILS presents with repeated infections in late childhood or adolescence. ELS more commonly presents in newborns as respiratory distress, cyanosis, or pneumonia [20].

In many cases of ILS, cystic structures are formed by dilated airways containing mucopurulent material. There is a strong association between ELS and CPAM type 2, present within the lesion [14]. As described above, BPS occasionally presents as a heterogeneous mass with a cystic component termed a "hybrid lesion" (BPS and CPAM Fig. 4.5); the CPAM is generally type 2 [21]. The key to differentiating between CPAM and BPS or hybrid lesions is detection of an aberrant artery. If there is an aberrant artery, CPAM is excluded [10].

On fetal US, ELS may be seen as early as 16 weeks' gestation and typically appears as a solid, well-defined, triangular, echogenic mass lesion (Fig. 4.6). Color Doppler may identify a feeding vessel arising from the aorta. If the sequestration is located infra-diaphragmatically, it may appear as an echogenic intra-abdominal mass masquerading as a suprarenal mass like a neuroblastoma [22].

Fetal MRI is also supportive in confirming the diagnosis of BPS and can also be used to estimate the volume and maturity of normal lung tissue. Another advantage of fetal MRI is evaluation of other associated disease such as CPAM (a hybrid lesion) and congenital diaphragmatic hernias, which are common with the extralobar type (50–60%) [20].

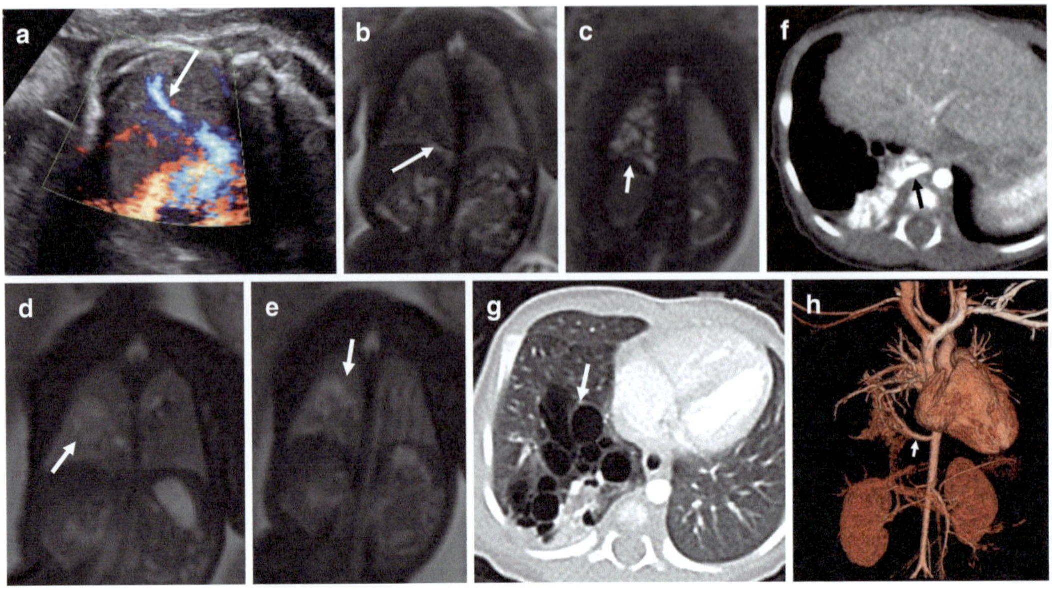

**Fig. 4.5** Hybrid lesion (bronchopulmonary sequestration and CPAM). Axial view of color Doppler fetal US (**a**) at 32 gestational weeks. Coronal fetal MRI at 31 gestational weeks (SSTSE sequence [**b**, **c**, **d**, **e**]), contrast-enhanced chest CT at 3 days old (**f**, **g**) and 3-DCT reconstruction (**h**). Color Doppler fetal US showed abnormal vascular structure arising from thoracic aorta (**a**, arrow) as an aberrant artery. Coronal view of SSTSE showed linear signal void structure as abnormal vascular structure in right lower lung (**b**, arrow). Bronchopulmonary sequestration with its aberrant artery was suspected. Otherwise, multiple cystic components were associated (**c**, **d**, e arrows). These appearances suggested hybrid lesion of bronchopulmonary sequestration and CPAM. Contrast-enhanced chest CT performed at 3 days old revealed obvious aberrant artery (**f**, **h**, arrow) and multiple lung cysts 8–10 mm in diameter on lung field window image (**g**, arrow). The patient underwent surgical operation and pathological specimen showed intralobar sequestration and terminal bronchiole with cystic dilatation. Diagnosis of hybrid lesion was established on pathological examination

Two different sequences are used for T2WI series in fetal MRI, namely, SSTSE and b-SSFP sequences. SSTSE is also called "HASTE" with Siemens MRI, and "SSFSE" with GE MRI. Aoki et al. evaluated the utility of a SSTSE Sequence as compared with b-SSFP [10].

SSTSE sequences reveal vessels as a dark signal due to the flow void phenomenon (Fig. 4.6). In contrast, on b-SSFP sequences, vessels appear bright, with the same signal intensity as background lung parenchyma. In their research series, the SSTSE sequence was superior to a b-SSFP sequence for clear visualization of the aberrant artery in BPS, regardless of the arterial diameter and background heterogeneity. A SSTSE sequence is essential for detecting aberrant arteries in the diagnosis of BPS on fetal MRI. Accuracy may not be affected by either arterial diameter or background heterogeneity [10].

## 4.6 Bronchial Atresia (BA)

BA consists of focal obliteration of the proximal segment of a bronchus with normal architecture of the distal lung. The airway obstruction impairs the elimination of the distally produced pulmonary fluid, causing fluid accumulation, expansion, and homogeneously increased echogenicity at antenatal US and high signal intensity on T2-weighted fetal MR images of the involved lung (Fig. 4.7). These prenatal imaging findings are nonspecific and may be also observed in other congenital lung malformations [1]. The exact cause of BA is not well known. Focal bronchial interruption seems to occur before birth. As the bronchial pattern is entirely normal distal to the site of stenosis, BA results from interruption of focal developmental of a lobar, segmental, or subsegmental bronchus and is associated with collateral alveolar fluid

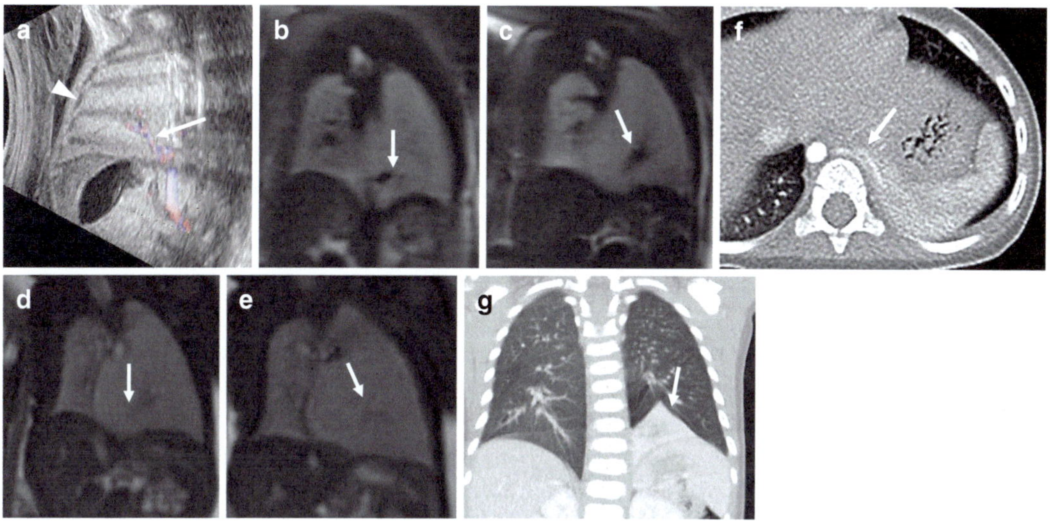

**Fig. 4.6** Bronchopulmonary sequestration (BPS): extralobar sequestration (ELS). Sagittal view of color Doppler fetal US (**a**) and coronal fetal MRI at 31 gestational weeks (SSTSE sequence [**b**, **c**] and b-SSFP sequence [**d**, **e**]), contrast-enhanced chest CT at 6 days old (**f**, **g**). Note distended left lower lung (**a**, arrowheads) with abnormal vascular structure (**a**, arrow) on color Doppler image. This vascular structure was diagnosed as an aberrant artery originating from the thoracic aorta. These characteristic findings suggest a diagnosis of BPS. SSTSE sequence fetal MRI clearly showed a low signal vascular structure (**b**, **c** arrow), which originated from the thoracic aorta. However, b-SSFP sequence could not demonstrate an aberrant artery (**d**, **e** arrow). On contrast-enhanced chest CT, note the aberrant artery (**f**, arrow) and no air in sequestrated lung parenchyma due to disconnection of airway (**g**, arrow). ELS was proved by surgical specimen

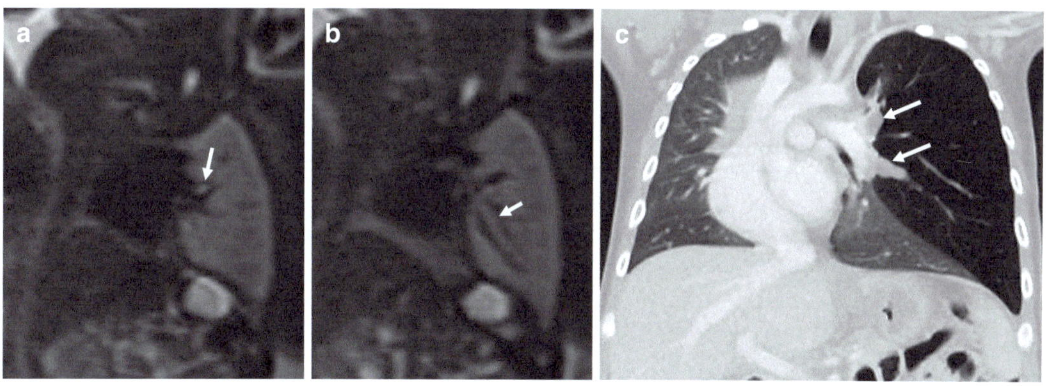

**Fig. 4.7** Bronchial atresia. Coronal fetal MRI at 28 gestational weeks (SSTSE sequence [**a**, **b**]), contrast-enhanced chest CT at 8 months old (**c**). Note expansion of left lung parenchyma without obvious cystic lesion on SSTSE images (**a**, **b**). Focal high signal spot was demonstrated at left pulmonary hilum (**a**, arrow), and this high signal structure was continuously demonstrated along with left pulmonary artery (**b**, arrow). Chest CT performed at 8 months revealed emphysematous change in left upper lobe and the bronchi filled with mucus and formation of a mucocele/bronchocele (**c**, arrow)

drift (not "fluid trapping" as in congenital lobar emphysema) through the surrounding lung parenchyma via the intra-alveolar pores of the Kohn, bronchoalveolar channels of Lambert, and intrabronchial channels [23]. The bronchi distal to the atresia become filled with mucus and may form a mucocele/bronchocele. The lung distal to the atretic bronchus develops normally but is overinflated due to collateral air drift with air trapping postnatally [24].

The typical prenatal imaging findings described in the literature for CPAM and BPS often allow a correct diagnosis of these abnormalities in utero. In contrast, BA is rarely diagnosed or even suggested before birth and not always recognized in neonates.

Alamo et al. distinguished two types of congenital BA by location, imaging findings and clinical evolution. The proximal type is located at the level of the main stem or the proximal lobar bronchi. Although extremely rare, it is often correctly identified in utero with a huge volume increase in the distal, involved lung, which appears homogeneously hyperechoic at US and hyperintense on T2WI MR images. In such cases, the bronchocele is a centrally located, fluid-filled tubular structure, is often observed and reflects dilatation of the bronchus distal to the atresia. Proximal atresia seems to affect the right lung predominantly [1].

The second type of BA, peripheral, is located at a segmental/subsegmental bronchial level. It may present as an isolated lesion or be associated with other anomalies in a complex malformation, mainly the microcystic type of CPAM.

The prenatal identification of BA in these cases is extremely difficult as the associated malformation usually shows typical imaging findings that may mask the atresia.

Bronchial dilation may also be present in peripheral BA, but it is rarely detected prospectively because of its small size [1].

## 4.7 Congenital Lobar Emphysema (CLE)

CLE refers to overexpansion of a pulmonary lobe occurring in an infant [14]. It usually involves the left upper or right middle lobes. On fetal US and MRI, CLE appears as a fluid-overloaded lung lobe. CLE may occur when transient mucus plug impaction, extrinsic compression by a mass lesion, or abnormalities of cartilage cause bronchial narrowing, and it usually involves the left upper or right middle lobes [23].

Fetal US may demonstrate gradually increasing or decreasing echogenicity of the fetal lung lesion [25]. MRI should differentiate CLE from micro-/macrocystic CPAM because of the homogeneity and intact lung structure with stretched hilar vessels [25]. BPS can also be differentiated from CLE by the presence of a systemic arterial supply. However, differentiation between CLE and BPS might be difficult due to the similar pathogenesis.

## 4.8 Congenital Bronchogenic Cyst

Congenital bronchogenic cysts are caused by abnormal budding from the ventral embryonic foregut along the tracheobronchial tree, which subsequently differentiates into a fluid-filled, blind-ending pouch that is typically located in the mediastinum near the tracheal carina [23]. Less commonly, cysts can occur within the lung parenchyma, pleura, or diaphragm [23]. The bronchogenic cyst walls are thin, are covered by respiratory epithelium, and contain mucinous material. Fetal MR imaging aids in determining the location of the suspected lesion. On fetal MRI, the cyst has markedly high intensity on T2WI, where there is a single cystic component [2]. Hyperechoic bronchogenic cysts might be more easily visualized with MRI than with US [4].

## 4.9 Summary

Compared with non-exposure, exposure to 1.5 Tesla MRI during any trimester of pregnancy was not associated with an increased risk of harm, either to the fetus or in early childhood. ACR-SPR guidelines suggest that fetal MRI is appropriate after 18 weeks' gestational age.

Congenital lung abnormalities (CLAs) are heterogeneous entities consisting of bronchopulmonary anomalies, vascular anomalies or a combination of these. The most common CLA is congenital pulmonary airway malformation (CPAM), followed by bronchopulmonary sequestration (BPS), bronchial atresia (BA), bronchogenic cyst and congenital lobar overinflation (CLO) or congenital lobar emphysema (CLE). Two different sequences of T2WI series, single-shot turbo spin echo (SSTSE) and balanced-steady state free precession (b-SSFP), are available for evaluation of lung parenchyma. The SSTSE sequence is essential for detecting aberrant arteries in the diagnosis of BPS on fetal MRI.

## References


1. Alamo L, Vial Y, Gengler C, Meuli R. Imaging findings of bronchial atresia in fetuses, neonates and infants. Pediatr Radiol. 2016;46:383–90.
2. Pacharn P, Kline-Fath B, Calvo-Garcia M, Linam LE, Rubio EI, Salisbury S, Brody AS. Congenital lung lesions: prenatal MRI and postnatal findings. Pediatr Radiol. 2013;43:1136–43.
3. Biyyam DR, Chapman T, Ferguson MR, Deutsch G, Dighe MK. Congenital lung abnormalities: embryologic features, prenatal diagnosis, and postnatal radiologic-pathologic correlation. Radiographics. 2010;30:1721–38.
4. Beydon BN, Larroquet M, Coulomb A, Jouannic J-M, le Pointe HD, Clément A, Garel C. Comparison between US and MRI in the prenatal assessment of lung malformations. Pediatr Radiol. 2013;43:685–96.
5. ACR–SPR practice parameter for th safe and optimal performance of fetal magnetic resonance imaging (MRI). https://www.acr.org/-/media/ACR/Files/Practice-Parameters/mr-fetal. Access date 23 September 2019.
6. Ray JG, Vermeulen MJ, Bharatha A, Montanera WJ, Park AL. Association between MRI exposure during pregnancy and fetal and childhood outcomes. JAMA. 2016;316:952–61.
7. Victoria T, Jaramillo D, Roberts TP, Zarnow D, Johnson AM, Delgado J, Rubesova E, Vossough A. Fetal magnetic resonance imaging: jumping from 1.5 to 3 tesla (preliminary experience). Pediatr Radiol. 2014;44:376–86.
8. Chartier AL, Bouvier MJ, McPherson DR, Stepenosky JE, Taysom DA. Marks RM. The safety of maternal and fetal MRI at 3T. AJR Am J Roentgenol. 2019;16:1–4.
9. Chapman T, Alazraki AL, Eklund MJ. A survey of pediatric diagnostic radiologists in North America: current practices in fetal magnetic resonance imaging. Pediatr Radiol. 2018;48:1924–35.
10. Aoki H, Miyazaki O, Okamoto R, Tsutsumi Y, Miyasaka M, Sago H, Kanamori Y, Yoshioka T, Nosaka S. Fetal MRI to assess an aberrant artery in Bronchopulmonary sequestration: the utility of a single-shot turbo spin Echo sequence. J Fetal Med. 2019;6:127–32.
11. Chavhan GB, Babyn PS, Jankharia BG, Cheng HL, Shroff MM. Steady- state MR imaging sequences: physics, classification, and clinical applications. Radiographics. 2008;28:1147–60.
12. Daltro P, Werner H, Gasparetto TD, Domingues RC, Rodrigues L, Marchiori E, Gasparetto EL. Congenital chest malformations: a multimodality approach with emphasis on fetal MR imaging. Radiographics. 2010;30:385–95.
13. Kuwashima S, Nishimura G, Iimura F, Kohno T, Watanabe H, Kohno A, Fujioka M. Low-intensity fetal lungs on MRI may suggest the diagnosis of pulmonary hypoplasia. Pediatr Radiol. 2001;31: 669–72.
14. Stocker JC, Husain AN. Cystic lesions of the lung in children: Classification and controversies. In K. Larsson editor. Chief; European respiratory. Monograph 39 2007, March. p. 1–20 Printed in UK.
15. Adzick NS, Harrison MR, Glick PL, Golbus MS, Anderson RL, Mahony BS, Callen PW, Hirsch JH, Luthy DA, Filly RA. Fetal cystic adenomatoid malformation: prenatal diagnosis and natural history. J Pediatr Surg. 1985;205:483–8.
16. Di Prima FA, Bellia A, Inclimona G, Grasso F, Teresa M, Cassaro MN. Antenatally diagnosed congenital cystic adenomatoid malformations (CCAM): research review. J Prenat Med. 2012;6:22–30.
17. Barth RA. Airway anomalies, lung and medias masses, and hydrothorax. In: Kline-Fath BM, Bulsa DI, Bahado-Singh RB, editors. Fundamental and advanced fetal imaging. 1st ed. Philadelphia: Walters Kluwer; 2015. p. 596–615.
18. Owada K, Miyazaki O, Matsuoka K, Sago H, Nosaka S. Unusual signal intensity of congenital pulmonary airway malformation on fetal magnetic resonance imaging. Pediatr Radiol. 2015;45:763–6.
19. Victoria T, Srinivasan AS, Pogoriler J, Kreiger PA, Laje P, Oliver ER, Danzer E, Johnson AM, Moldenhauer JS, Peranteau WH, Adzick S. The rare solid fetal lung lesion with T2-hypointense components: prenatal imaging findings with postnatal pathological correlation. Pediatr Radiol. 2018;48: 1556–66.
20. Radiopedia Pulmonary sequestration. https://radiopaedia.org/articles/pulmonary-sequestration?lang=us. Accessed 23 September 2019.
21. Recio Rodríguez M, Martínez de Vega V, Cano Alonso R, Carrascoso Arranz J, Martínez Ten P, Pérez Pedregosa J. MR imaging of thoracic abnormalities in the fetus. Radiographics. 2012;32:E305–21.
22. Kalenahalli KV, Garg N, Goolahally LN, Reddy SP, Iyengar J. Infradiaphragmatic extralobar pulmonary sequestration: masquerading as suprarenal mass. J Clin Neonatol. 2013;2:146–8.
23. Liu PY, Lin YL, Chen SC. Fetal magnetic resonance imaging of congenital chest malformations: a pictorial review. J Radiol Sci. 2013;38:119–27.
24. Radiopedia Bronchial atresia. https://radiopaedia.org/articles/bronchial-atresia?lang=us. Accessed 9 November 2019.
25. Liu YP, Shih SL. Congenital lobar emphysema: appearance on fetal MRI. Pediatr Radiol. 2008;38:1264.

# 5 Perinatal Care for Severe Congenital Pulmonary Airway Malformation

Yushi Ito

**Abstract**

Congenital pulmonary airway malformation (CPAM) is one of the most common lung lesions identified via fetal ultrasonography. Although the lesion either regresses throughout the pregnancy or remains unchanged and leads to favorable outcomes in the majority of cases, fetuses with hydrops fetalis and severe mediastinal shift are at risk of intrauterine demise or neonatal death. Thoracoamniotic shunting between the large cyst and amniotic space or antenatal steroids is the treatment of choice for the management of fetuses with CPAM accompanied with hydrops fetalis. These interventions in utero affect the treatment strategy of resuscitation and management immediately after birth as well as the outcomes. Thus, newborns with severe CPAM who were subjected to thoracoamniotic shunting in utero should be planned with emergency surgery strategies immediately after birth with the cooperation of obstetricians, surgeons, neonatologists, and anesthesiologists.

**Keywords**

Congenital pulmonary airway malformation (CPAM) · Fetal ultrasonography · Macrocystic type · Microcystic type Mixed type · CPAM volume ratio (CVR) Thoracoamniotic shunt · Antenatal steroid Emergency surgery strategy · Bronchial atresia (BA) · Pulmonary sequestration

## 5.1 Introduction

Congenital pulmonary airway malformation (CPAM) is one of the most common lung lesions identified via fetal ultrasonography. Currently, every 1 in 12,000–15,000 live births experiences CPAM [1, 2] . Recent studies have defined the natural course of this condition. The condition rapidly progresses between 20–25 weeks of gestation, plateaus off at 25 weeks, and regresses after 29 weeks [3–6]. Although the lesion either regresses through the pregnancy or remains unchanged and leads to favorable outcomes in majority of cases, fetuses with hydrops fetalis and severe mediastinal shift are at risk of intrauterine demise or neonatal death [3, 7–12].

To obtain an accurate picture of the condition and fetuses at risk for adverse outcomes, several parameters obtained through fetal sonographic measurements have been established [2, 13, 14] .

Y. Ito (✉)
Division of Neonatology, Center for Maternal-Fetal, Neonatal and Reproductive Medicine, National Center for Child Health and Development, Tokyo, Japan
e-mail: itoh-yu@ncchd.go.jp





H. Sago et al. (eds.), *Congenital Cystic Lung Disease*, https://doi.org/10.1007/978-981-15-5175-8_5

A CPAM volume ratio (CVR) of $\geq 1.6$ with a sensitivity of 75%, a positive predictive value of 60%, and a negative predictive value of 98% are considered risk factors for the development of hydrops fetalis. Meanwhile, fetuses with a CVR cutoff of $<1.0$ are less likely to experience adverse outcomes and are predicted to be asymptomatic at birth with a probability of almost 100% [14, 15].

Thoracoamniotic shunting between the large cyst and amniotic space or antenatal steroids has been the treatment of choice for CPAM accompanied with hydrops fetalis and has led to the improvement of hydrops and diminished lesions. These interventions in utero affect the treatment strategy of resuscitation and management immediately after birth as well as the outcomes.

In this chapter, the management of neonates with severe CPAM after birth will be described.

## 5.2 Prenatal Management and Clinical Course

Perinatal management [9] is focused on the prolongation of the pregnancy period and the mitigation of compression to the mediastinum through reduction of the size of CPAM lesion. Presence of fetal edema and size of cystic lesion are assessed via fetal ultrasonography. According to ultrasonographic findings, cystic lesions are classified into macrocystic type (cyst size of φ5 mm or more) and microcystic type (less than φ5 mm) [16]. Fetal magnetic resonance imaging (MRI) is also performed to evaluate the shape and size of cystic lesions, the degree of mediastinal shift, and the condition of healthy lungs [17]. The size of the cystic lesion is monitored over time by CVR [4].

### 5.2.1 Classification Based on Pathological Findings and Fetal Sonographic Appearance

The original classification of CPAM proposed by Stocker [16] includes three types based on pathological findings. Type 1 lesions comprise single or multiple large cysts (>2 cm in diameter) that result in mediastinal herniation frequently. In these lesions, the cysts are lined by ciliated pseudostratified columnar epithelium, and the cyst walls contain prominent smooth muscle and elastic tissue. Mucus-producing cells are present in approximately one-third of the cases, and cartilage is rarely found in the cyst wall. Relatively normal alveoli may be seen between the cysts. Type 2 lesions are composed of multiple small cysts (<1 cm in diameter) that are lined by ciliated cuboidal/columnar epithelium. Structures resembling respiratory bronchioles and distended alveoli are present between the epithelium-lined cysts. Mucous cells and cartilage are not present, and striated muscle fibers may be seen rarely. Type 3 lesions are large, bulky, non-cystic lesions that produce mediastinal shift macroscopically. These lesions comprise smaller cystic lesions (<2 mm in diameter). Histologically, bronchiole-like structures are lined by ciliated cuboidal epithelium and separated by masses of alveolus-sized structures lined by non-ciliated cuboidal epithelium. The revised classification proposed by Stocker [18, 19] adds two new types, type 0 and type 4, to the original classification. Type 0, including hypoplastic lungs composed of bronchiole-like structures with extensive cartilage tissue, was previously defined as acinar dysplasia [20, 21]. Type 4 lesions are single large cysts in peripheral zones of the lobe or near the pleura. The wall of the cyst is thin and lined by alveolar epithelium-like epithelial cells.

Type 1 lesions account for 50% of postnatal cases of CPAM and are usually associated with a favorable outcome. Conversely, type 2 lesions, which account for 40% of postnatal cases of CPAM, are associated frequently with congenital anomalies including renal agenesis or dysgenesis, truncus arteriosus and tetralogy of Fallot, jejunal atresia, diaphragmatic hernia, hydrocephalus, and skeletal anomalies [16]. The prognosis of type 3 CPAMs, which are typically large, homogeneous, microcystic masses that account for only 10% of cases, is variable; however, severe cases of type 3 CPAMs develop hydrops and present with cardiorespiratory compromise in the newborn [22].

Based on the fetal ultrasonographic findings, Adzick et al. have proposed a modification of Stocker's classification [22] by characterizing CPAMs into the macrocystic and microcystic types according to the fetal sonographic findings. In the proposed classification, macrocystic CPAMs are defined by the presence of single or multiple cysts that are ≥5 mm in diameter. In contrast, microcystic CPAMs are characterized as more solid and bulky comprising cysts that are <5 mm in diameter. Sonographically, macrocystic lesions appear as fluid-filled cysts whereas microcystic lesions are observed as solid structures with almost homogeneous appearance [22]. Fetuses with very large CPAMs (CVR ≥ 1.6) that cause a mediastinal shift toward the healthy side and a diaphragm shift toward the abdominal side tend to develop hydrops fetalis due to mediastinal compression, which can result in cardiac failure. Large microcystic lesions are at increased risk for the development of hydrops and pulmonary hypoplasia, leading to high mortality rate [1, 3, 22].

Based on their analysis of 170 cases with CPAM, Cavoretto et al. [9] reported that microcystic, macrocystic, and mixed lesions were present in 90 (52.9%), 38 (22.4%), and 42 (24.7%) cases, respectively, and that 9 (5.3%) cases developed hydrops fetalis.

### 5.2.2 Evaluation of Cystic Lesion Size Using Fetal Ultrasonography

Developed by Cromblehome et al., the CVR creates a gestational age-corrected volume ratio for prognostic predication [4, 23]. Fetuses with a CVR of ≥1.6 were found to be at increased risk for developing hydrops fetalis. A recent study of 64 cases of lung lesions found that a CVR of ≥1.6 had a sensitivity of 75%, a positive predictive value of 60%, and a negative predictive value of 98% for the detection of hydrops fetalis [14, 15]. The same study also proposed that a CVR cutoff of <1.0 in infants is indicative of a less likely presence of adverse outcomes, predicting a probability of almost 100% absence of symptoms at birth [14, 15].

### 5.2.3 Treatment of Fetuses with CPAM

The cystic lesion size is consistently monitored on the basis of the CVR. All fetuses are followed up using ultrasonography if there is no fetal edema and the CVR is <1.6. In contrast, for fetuses with a macrocystic/mixed type lesion with a CVR of ≥1.6 and large cysts (maximum diameter: ≥20 mm) or with a microcystic type lesion with a CVR of ≥1.6 and fluid retention in the body cavity with/without fetal edema, fetal treatment is considered up to 34 weeks of gestation. Cyst puncture is performed first, after which reduction in the large cystic cavity size is confirmed in macrocystic/mixed type lesions with large cysts (largest diameter: ≥20 mm). Second, thoracoamniotic shunting [9, 24, 25] is offered to cases when fluid retention in the cyst occurs soon after the cyst puncture. For fetuses with microcystic type lesions whose CVRs are ≥1.6 and/or who develop hydrops fetalis, antenatal maternal betamethasone (12 mg intramuscular injection for 2 days) is administered [26, 27]; however, administration of antenatal maternal steroid therapy is still debatable because most of the microcystic CPAM tends to regress spontaneously after a growth peak at approximately 25–28 weeks of gestation [3].

### 5.2.4 Response to Fetal Treatment and Condition Just Before Birth

Ninety-five percent of fetuses with CPAM diagnosed in utero do not develop hydrops fetalis and survive throughout the pregnancy; further, they are expected to be born in good condition. Cavoretto [9] recently reported that 161 of 170 fetuses with CPAM did not develop hydrops fetalis but 9 did. Of the 161 fetuses that did not develop hydrops fetalis, 6 with macrocystic CPAM were offered a thoracoamniotic shunt, and all those infants survived. Of nine CPAM fetuses with hydrops, four had macrocystic lesions, two had mixed lesions, and three had microcystic lesions. Three and two fetuses with macrocystic and mixed lesions, respectively, were offered a thoracoamniotic shunt. One hydropic fetus with a mixed lesion with shunting died in utero, but the other four hydropic fetuses with shunting survived.

At our perinatal center, 83 fetuses were diagnosed with CPAM between May 2002 and September 2017 [28]. Of 51 fetuses who had macrocystic lesions, 24 had a large cyst (diameter: ≥20 mm), and 13 of them were offered thoracoamniotic shunt. Of 26 fetuses that were diagnosed as having microcystic lesions, seven were given an antenatal steroid. Twenty-two fetuses with CPAM who had fluid retention in their body cavity (ascites or pleural effusion) and/or edema were offered thoracoamniotic shunt or administered antenatal steroids. Of 13 fetuses with hydrops fetalis, 2 were born without fluid retention in the body cavity and edema, 5 were born with only fluid retention in the body cavity without edema, and 6 were born with fluid retention in the body cavity with edema. However, of 13 fetuses with CPAM and hydrops fetalis, 8 unfortunately died in the neonatal period.

Over all, approximately 90% of the fetuses with severe CPAM type 1 to whom thoracoamniotic shunting was offered survived throughout the study. On the other hand, about 45% of CPAM fetuses with hydrops fetalis remain hydropic until birth, even when treatments were applied in the fetal period. Table 5.1 shows the classification of fetuses with CPAM in severity of condition.

**Table 5.1** Classification of fetuses with CPAM as per the severity of condition

| Stage | Size of CPAM | Original hydrops and distress before fetal treatment | Fetal treatment | Final hydrops and distress before birth |
|---|---|---|---|---|
| F1 | CVR < 1.6 (CVR < 1.0) | No | No | No |
| F2 | CVR ≥ 1.6 or large cystic lesion (max φ ≥ 20 mm) | Yes or no | Yes | No |
| F3 | CVR ≥ 1.6 or large cystic lesion (max φ ≥ 20 mm) | Yes | Yes or no | Yes or fetal death |

## 5.3 Management of Neonates with CPAM at Birth and Infancy

To clearly comprehend the clinical course and estimated diagnosis and to discuss immediate neonatal resuscitation and treatment after birth, in advance, a clinical conference for fetuses with severe CPAM will be held in coordination with all departments in charge prior to the birth of the child. If no maternal and fetal problems are found upon assessment, delivery is planned at 37–38 weeks of gestation. For cases in which fetal treatment (thoracoamniotic shunt) has been performed and in whom respiratory distress is expected to develop immediately after birth by rapid dilatation of the large cystic lesion with inspired air trapped in large macrocystic CPAM (type 1) and mixed type (type 2), emergency surgery strategy is applied. The fetuses are delivered by elective Caesarean section and neonatal resuscitation should be performed inside the operating room for immediate shift to emergency surgery strategy.

The other neonates with CPAM who are not expected respiratory distress rightly after birth are resuscitated following the guidelines of the Neonatal Resuscitation Program basically.

In fetuses with large microcystic CPAM (CVR of ≥1.6), emergency surgery strategy is avoided and care with the help of a ventilator, inhaled nitric oxide, and catecholamine at the NICU is administered to stabilize the condition first. If respiratory failure is not improved after the stabilization in NICU, surgical resection is then considered to exert pressure via the large CPAM on the healthy lung.

Infants who develop respiratory failure a couple of days after birth are urged to undergo surgery to resect the involved lung in case of mixed and microcystic lesions.

Constant monitoring and follow-up of all neonates with CPAM, including those with no respiratory distress in the NICU, on their respiratory condition and growth at the outpatient clinic by the pediatric pulmonologist and surgeon should be performed after discharge.

### 5.3.1 Emergency Surgery Strategy

Emergency surgery strategy is administered to neonates with severe CPAM whose respiratory distress is expected to follow immediately after birth by immediate dilatation of large cystic lesion with inspired air trapped in large macrocystic CPAM (type 1), to whom thoracoamniotic shunt was offered. Neonatal resuscitation should be performed inside the operating room for immediate shift to emergency surgery strategy when the need arises. The emergency surgery strategy is planned based on careful coordination with the obstetrician, midwife, neonatologist, NICU nurse, surgeon, anesthesiologist, operating room nurse, medical engineer, etc. Everything that the pregnant women and her family need to know about neonatal resuscitation and emergent surgery right after birth is explained and provided; written consent is obtained in advance, and consent for emergent blood transfusion with type O blood to the neonate is also obtained.

### 5.3.2 Points and Pitfalls of Each Department's Role in Emergency Surgery Strategy for Neonates with Severe CPAM

#### 5.3.2.1 Department of Obstetrics for Fetal Medicine

The obstetric team is responsible for fetal diagnosis, management, and delivery. When need for emergency surgery of the neonate arises immediately after birth, the obstetrician should opt for a cesarean section.

With regards to large prepartum cysts and the presence of mediastinal displacement regardless of fetal treatment, no consensus has been reached as to whether the fluid in it should be aspirated through cyst puncture and whether the large cyst should be diminished just before delivery. Researchers do not recommend this because a collapsed large cyst through puncture and aspiration just before birth tends to re-expand immediately after birth through inspiratory air, thereby leading to compression of the heart as well as circulatory collapse within few seconds. In fact, reportedly, a newborn had cardiac arrest few seconds after delivery following prepuncture and aspiration of fluid in the large cyst just before delivery and needed resuscitation by chest compression and ECMO after resection of CPAM immediately after birth. In contrast, infants with large cysts who did not undergo prepuncture and aspiration just before delivery can breathe and keep their heart rate and blood pressure stable in several tens of minutes without circulatory collapse even with low-oxygen saturation levels. Presumably, it is because it will not be easy and take several tens of minutes to replace the fluid in the large cyst with air; however, it will be easier and faster to expand the collapsed cyst and not a fluid-filled cyst using inspiratory air.

#### 5.3.2.2 Department of Neonatology

The Department of Neonatology is responsible for provision of immediate resuscitation right after birth. Neonatal resuscitation should be performed in the operating room for a swift shift in emergent surgery strategy when the need arises. The important thing to remember in neonatal resuscitation for CPAM-affected neonates is avoiding positive-pressure tidal ventilation and supporting spontaneous breathing as much as possible to be able to gain enough time until air enters the cyst filled with lung water and the cyst is expandable by inspiratory air.

If bradycardia occurs after birth, bag–valve–mask ventilation should be performed, but if bag–valve–mask ventilation also does not suffice, the trachea should be intubated and shift to emergency surgery strategy should be made. Cardiopulmonary resuscitation, including chest compression, should be performed when necessary. After intubation, positive-pressure ventilation should be maintained with minimum inspiratory pressure, and the infant should be kept on ventilator with the SIMV and HFOV modes at the resuscitation site. To avoid tidal ventilation with high inspiratory pressure, the infant should be administered CPAP with PEEP of 5 cm $H_2O$ if possible; otherwise, the infant should be kept on the HFOV mode. Together with managing airway and breathing, at least one peripheral intravenous line or umbilical line should be obtained and emergency surgery strategy should be considered. The goal here is to maintain the heart rate rather than increase oxygen saturation; further, the anesthesiologist should be informed and take over the respiratory management when venous lines for drip infusion are secured.

If the neonate does not show severe respiratory distress within several minutes after birth, chest X-ray should be obtained to evaluate the dilatation of large cystic lesion by respiration and the neonates should be observed closely inside the operating room in several tens of minutes to decide whether emergency surgery is indicated or not.

#### 5.3.2.3 Department of Anesthesia

Anesthesiologists are responsible for collaborating information with obstetricians, neonatologists, and pediatric surgeons in advance and maintained on standby for emergency surgery. Basically, they are to keep the neonate under spontaneous breathing and avoid high positive pressure ventilation. Tracheal intubation should be performed right before skin incision by the surgeon. To avoid the possibility of closed cavity expansion, usage of sevoflurane as a volatile anesthetic agent and narcotics, such as fentanyl, should be considered.

#### 5.3.2.4 Department of Surgery

Surgeons are divided into two teams: an operating team and a roundabout team. The operating team should be ready on standby at the start of the cesarean section in case surgery is needed. The medical staff of the roundabout team on the other hand prepares to place the patient in a side immediately after neonatal resuscitation in case of emergency surgery strategy. Time should not be spent on side preparation and disinfection alone. If mediastinum compression and circulatory collapse occur, release of the pressure of the expanded cyst through opening of the chest cavity and cyst through fenestration or the extrathoracic cavity should be performed immediately. Breathing and circulation improve soon after opening chest cavity and large cyst, and this stage is particularly rapid. This part of management is crucial in critical infants.

In several cases, there is not enough time to perform chest CT imaging, and there is only little positional information on the lung lobes affected by fetal MRI or plain chest X-ray alone. If the lesion extends over multiple lobes after thoracotomy, only the lobe of the primary lesion may be removed and small lesions may remain.

In newborns, a few split lobe failures of the lung may be present, and it is often easy to comprehend the arteriovenous system positioning of the lung. Hence, it is important that the diseased lung lobes be shrunk by creating an opening on the cysts to avoid restriction of the visual field by a large cystic lesion. As for bronchial treatment, because the bronchium is thin and soft, the sweet technique is not forcibly performed, and no particular problem occurs even in the simple penetration and ligation methods. The remaining lung lobes are small and immature due to compression of giant cysts, and air leaks often close spontaneously; hence, sticking to repair may rather promote air leaks.

## 5.4 Management of Patients with CPAM in Infancy and Childhood

Patients with severe CPAM are continuously monitored by neonatologists in the NICU. Persistent pulmonary hypertension of the newborn resulting from emergency surgery stress immediately after birth and hypoplasia of the residual lung can occur, and several infants need nitric oxide therapy after a couple of days.

Some infants who develop respiratory failure in a couple of days after birth in the NICU will have to undergo surgery to excise the affected lung.

All neonates with CPAM should be closely observed after birth using chest X-ray and CT scan to evaluate changes in cystic lesions, if any, in the NICU.

Meanwhile, newborns that do not have respiratory distress should still be followed up and checked for respiratory condition and growth at the outpatient clinic by the corresponding pediatric pulmonologist and surgeon. At around 9 months, these infants with CPAM should have contrast CT, bronchoscopy, bronchography, and angiography performed; elective surgery up to age 1 is dependent on the clinical diagnosis obtained.

Table 5.2 shows the classification of infants with CPAM based on the clinical course after birth, whereas Table 5.3 shows the management for neonates with CPAM in the perinatal period.

**Table 5.2** Classification of neonates with CPAM in the clinical course after birth

| Stage | Treatment in neonatal period | Timing of surgery | Outcome |
|---|---|---|---|
| N1 | No treatment | Before 1 years old | Good |
| N2 | Respiratory support | 2–6 days or 1–3 weeks after birth | Good |
| N3 | Respiratory support immediately after birth | 0–3 hours after birth | Good |
| N4 | Respiratory support immediately after birth | Not indicated or dies after surgery | Poor |

Even after discharge from the NICU, these patients will belong to the high-risk group of pulmonary diseases in infancy and childhood. Hama et al. in their study [29] reported a high incidence of pulmonary infection in infants with severe CPAM who needed partial lung resection surgery in the neonatal periods and recommended that these infants with severe CPAM be given palivizumab to prevent further RS virus infection.

## 5.5 Discussion and Future Perspective

Congenital cystic lung disease includes diseases such as CPAM, bronchial atresia (BA), intralobar pulmonary sequestration (ILS), extralobar pulmonary sequestration (ELS), etc. Diagnosis is not easy; contrast CT, bronchoscopy, bronchography, and angiography are performed prior together with the pathological diagnosis of a resected specimen before a final diagnosis is reached. On the other hand, with fetal diagnosis, although limited to fetal ultrasound and MRI, the degree of severity depends on whether the

**Table 5.3** Fetal and neonatal management and clinical classifications

| Stocher's classification | Evalustion of lesion size (CVR>1.6 and/or hydrops fetslis) | Fetal treatment | Hydrops at birth | Fetal classification | Management at birth and infancy | Neonatal classification |
|---|---|---|---|---|---|---|
| Type 1 (Macrocystic type) | Yes (diameter of largest cyst ≥ 20 mm) | Cyst puncture/ thoracoamniotic shunt | Yes | F3 | Early surgery immediately after birth | N3 |
| | | | No | F2 | | |
| | No | None | | F1 | Observation and delayed surgery | N1 |
| Type 2 (Mixed type) | Yes | Cyst puncture/ thoracoamniotic shunt Antenatal steroid | Yes | F3 | Early surgery immediately after birth | N3 |
| | | | No | F2 | Consider surgery after stabilization | N2 |
| | No | None | | F1 | Observation and delayed surgery | N1 |
| Type 3 (Microcystic type) | Yes | Antenatal steroid | Yes | F3 | Early surgery immediately after birth | N3 or N4 |
| | | | | | Consider surgery after stabilization | N2 or N4 |
| | | | No | F2 | | N2 or N1 |
| | No | None | | F1 | Observation and delayed surgery | N1 |

lesion is macrocystic or microcystic and how much the surrounding organs are compressed; therefore, the method of fetal and perinatal treatment will be decided based on this limited information.

In our analysis [30, 31] of 105 cases in which lung resection was performed between March 2002 and August 2012 at our perinatal center, 52 were diagnosed in the fetal period. Fifty percent had CPAM up on the fetal diagnosis, 25% BA, and 25% pulmonary sequestration. Fetal treatment was performed in 20 cases, 12 (60%) of which had fetal hydrops fetalis. Of the 23 patients who underwent surgery during the neonatal period, 16 had CPAM (69%), 5 had ELS (22%), and 2 had BA (9%). Unfortunately, six cases did not survive, and one died after fetal thoracotomy, another died before surgery, and four died after neonatal surgery. The final diagnoses at death were CPAM type 1 in three cases, CPAM type 3 in two, and ELS in one. All cases that did not survive had similar characteristics, including preterm birth, low birth weight, hydrops fetalis, and high CVR value. On the other hand, the survival rate of the 12 severe cases with hydrops fetalis was 50%, thereby suggesting poor prognosis in infants with severe CPAM.

The pathogenesis of congenital cystic lung disease is still not clearly understood. "Malformation sequence" occurs when bronchial closure occurs first as a developmental abnormality, resulting in various patterns of lesions depending on the timing, site, and degree of the occlusion. Clinically, there is no definite theory as to whether BA is an etiology of congenital cystic lung disease or an independent disease. CPAM and BA had different clinical features when examined from the fetal stage. That is, there are severe cases in which a large number of CPAMs are diagnosed in the fetus and treatment for the fetus is required, and most of the cases that did not survive with cystic lung lesion had CPAMs. Even if CPAMs are not diagnosed in the fetal stage, cases can still develop with respiratory disorder early in life and will require diagnosis and surgery. On the other hand, some studies have reported cases of fetal diagnosis of BA; however, the number of cases with BA was approximately 50% of that of CPAM, and there were few cases in the fetal stage and no dead cases with BA. Most neonates with BA are asymptomatic after birth; thus, surgery requirement during the neonatal period is rare. Meanwhile, most infants with BA are diagnosed through the occurrence of pneumonia in childhood and planed surgery.

Academically, the distinction between CPAM and BA is still under debate, but the factors to be considered with management for fetuses with cystic lung lesion are the morphological size of the lesion and compression on the surrounding organs. Fetal cyst puncture and thoracoamniotic shunting can be performed to reduce macrocystic lesions, whereas maternal steroid administration or natural regression can be used for microcystic lesions. Infants with severe CPAM can be saved by planning emergency surgery immediately after birth. However, for cases with hydrops fetalis as well as those with preterm birth and low birth weight accompanied with lung hypoplasia, further improvement of treatment strategies is crucial.

## References

1. Adzick NS, Harrison MR. Management of the fetus with a cystic adenomatoid malformation. World J Surg. 1993;17(3):342–9.
2. Ehrenberg-Buchner S, Stapf AM, Berman DR, Drongowski RA, Mychaliska GB, Treadwell MC, et al. Fetal lung lesions: can we start to breathe easier? Am J Obstet Gynecol. 2013;208(2):151. e1-7
3. Adzick NS, Harrison MR, Crombleholme TM, Flake AW, Howell LJ. Fetal lung lesions: management and outcome. Am J Obstet Gynecol. 1998;179(4):884–9.
4. Crombleholme TM, Coleman B, Hedrick H, Liechty K, Howell L, Flake AW, et al. Cystic adenomatoid malformation volume ratio predicts outcome in prenatally diagnosed cystic adenomatoid malformation of the lung. J Pediatr Surg. 2002;37(3):331–8.
5. Kunisaki SM, Barnewolt CE, Estroff JA, Ward VL, Nemes LP, Fauza DO, et al. Large fetal congenital cystic adenomatoid malformations: growth trends and patient survival. J Pediatr Surg. 2007;42(2):404–10.
6. Wilson RD, Hedrick HL, Liechty KW, Flake AW, Johnson MP, Bebbington M, et al. Cystic adenomatoid malformation of the lung: review of genetics, prenatal diagnosis, and in utero treatment. Am J Med Genet A. 2006;140(2):151–5.
7. Baird R, Puligandla PS, Laberge JM. Congenital lung malformations: informing best practice. Semin Pediatr Surg. 2014;23(5):270–7.

8. Bunduki V, Ruano R, da Silva MM, Miguelez J, Miyadahira S, Maksoud JG, et al. Prognostic factors associated with congenital cystic adenomatoid malformation of the lung. Prenat Diagn. 2000;20(6):459–64.
9. Cavoretto P, Molina F, Poggi S, Davenport M, Nicolaides KH. Prenatal diagnosis and outcome of echogenic fetal lung lesions. Ultrasound Obstet Gynecol. 2008;32(6):769–83.
10. Rice HE, Estes JM, Hedrick MH, Bealer JF, Harrison MR, Adzick NS. Congenital cystic adenomatoid malformation: a sheep model of fetal hydrops. J Pediatr Surg. 1994;29(5):692–6.
11. Thorpe-Beeston JG, Nicolaides KH. Cystic adenomatoid malformation of the lung: prenatal diagnosis and outcome. Prenat Diagn. 1994;14(8):677–88.
12. Vu L, Tsao K, Lee H, Nobuhara K, Farmer D, Harrison M, et al. Characteristics of congenital cystic adenomatoid malformations associated with nonimmune hydrops and outcome. J Pediatr Surg. 2007;42(8):1351–6.
13. Hadchouel A, Benachi A, Revillon Y, Rousseau V, Martinovic J, Verkarre V, et al. Factors associated with partial and complete regression of fetal lung lesions. Ultrasound Obstet Gynecol. 2011;38(1):88–93.
14. Yong PJ, Von Dadelszen P, Carpara D, Lim K, Kent N, Tessier F, et al. Prediction of pediatric outcome after prenatal diagnosis and expectant antenatal management of congenital cystic adenomatoid malformation. Fetal Diagn Ther. 2012;31(2):94–102.
15. Hellmund A, Berg C, Geipel A, Bludau M, Heydweiller A, Bachour H, et al. Prenatal diagnosis and evaluation of Sonographic predictors for intervention and adverse outcome in congenital pulmonary airway malformation. PLoS One. 2016;11(3):e0150474.
16. Stocker JT, Madewell JE, Drake RM. Congenital cystic adenomatoid malformation of the lung. Classification and morphologic spectrum. Hum Pathol. 1977;8(2):155–71.
17. Shirota C, Tainaka T, Nakane T, Tanaka Y, Hinoki A, Sumida W, et al. Usefulness of fetal magnetic resonance imaging for postnatal management of congenital lung cysts: prediction of probability for emergency surgery. BMC Pediatr. 2018;18(1):105.
18. Stocker JT. Congenital pulmonary airway malformation: a new name and expanded classification of congenital cystic adenomatoid malformation of the lung. Histopathology. 2002;41(suppl. 2):424–31.
19. Stocker JT. Cystic lung disease in infants and children. Fetal Pediatr Pathol. 2009;28(4):155–84.
20. Davidson LA, Batman P, Fagan DG. Congenital acinar dysplasia: a rare cause of pulmonary hypoplasia. Histopathology. 1998;32(1):57–9.
21. Rutledge JC, Jensen P. Acinar dysplasia: a new form of pulmonary maldevelopment. Hum Pathol. 1986;17(12):1290–3.
22. Adzick NS, Harrison MR, Glick PL, Golbus MS, Anderson RL, Mahony BS, et al. Fetal cystic adenomatoid malformation: prenatal diagnosis and natural history. J Pediatr Surg. 1985;20(5):483–8.
23. Adzick NS, Flake AW, Crombleholme TM. Management of congenital lung lesions. Semin Pediatr Surg. 2003;12(1):10–6.
24. Grethel EJ, Wagner AJ, Clifton MS, Cortes RA, Farmer DL, Harrison MR, et al. Fetal intervention for mass lesions and hydrops improves outcome: a 15-year experience. J Pediatr Surg. 2007;42(1):117–23.
25. Nitta H, Taira Y, Kinjo T, Chinen Y, Masamoto H, Sanabe N, et al. Fetal Thoracoamniotic shunting in a case of congenital pulmonary airway malformations with Hydrops Fetalis. AJP Rep. 2017;7(3):e185–e7.
26. Peranteau WH, Wilson RD, Liechty KW, Johnson MP, Bebbington MW, Hedrick HL, et al. Effect of maternal betamethasone administration on prenatal congenital cystic adenomatoid malformation growth and fetal survival. Fetal Diagn Ther. 2007;22(5):365–71.
27. Tsao K, Hawgood S, Vu L, Hirose S, Sydorak R, Albanese CT, et al. Resolution of hydrops fetalis in congenital cystic adenomatoid malformation after prenatal steroid therapy. J Pediatr Surg. 2003;38(3):508–10.
28. Sugibayashi R. Treatment and perinatal prognosis of congenital cystic lung disease from the viewpoint of fetal diagnosis. J Jpn Soc Perinatal Neonatal Med. 2019;54(suppl):16–7.
29. Hama I, Takahashi S, Nakamura T, Ito Y, Kawasaki K, Sago H. Risk of respiratory syncytial virus infection in infants with congenital cystic lung disease. Pediatr Int. 2015;57(2):253–7.
30. Watanabe T, Amari S, Ohno M, Tahara K, Takezoe T, Fuchimoto Y, et al. Initial management to perinatal emergency: points and pitfalls for fetus and newborn Newborn disease. How to manage accurately; Congenital cystic lung disease. Perinatal Medicine (Tokyo). 2015:933–6.
31. Watanabe T, Ohno M, Tahara K, Tomonaga K, Fuchimoto Y, Fujino A, et al. An investigation on clinical differences between congenital pulmonary airway malformation and bronchial atresia. J Pediatr Surg. 2018;53(12):2390–3.

# 6 Postnatal Imaging Diagnosis of Congenital Cystic Lung Disease

Kumiko Nozawa

**Abstract**

Congenital cystic lung diseases (CCLD) include several diseases, such as congenital bronchial atresia, congenital lobar emphysema, congenital pulmonary airway malformation, bronchopulmonary sequestration and bronchogenic cyst. Prenatal diagnosis of congenital lung diseases is widespread and postnatal imaging diagnosis of CCLD is important for patient management and treatment decisions. It is necessary to know their radiological manifestations, especially parenchymal abnormalities included cysts and air-trapping, vascular supply and drainage of the lesions and bronchial abnormalities, to appropriate diagnosis. Radiographs play a role in the detection and initial postnatal imaging evaluation in clinically suspected CCLD, and CT and MRI are required for confirmation of diagnosis and preoperative evaluation of surgical lesions.

**Keywords**

Congenital cystic lung disease (CCLD)
Congenital pulmonary airway malformation (CPAM) · Postnatal imaging
Bronchopulmonary sequestration · Extralobar sequestration (ELS) · Intralobar sequestration (ILS) · Bronchial atresia (BA) · Congenital lobar emphysema (CLE) · Computed tomography (CT)

K. Nozawa (✉)
Department of Radiology, Kanagawa Children's Medical Center, Kanagawa, Yokohama, Japan
e-mail: knozawa@kcmc.jp

## 6.1 Introduction

Postnatal imaging diagnosis of congenital cystic lung disease (CCLD) is important for patient management and treatment decisions. CT is the most useful modality because of the need to assess both lung parenchyma and vascular structure. We review the typical radiological findings of CCLD and the role of diagnostic modalities.

## 6.2 Diagnostic Modalities

### 6.2.1 Chest Radiography

Chest radiography is the most frequent examination performed to evaluate the respiratory system and thoracic diseases in pediatric patients, and usually it is the initial imaging modality for patients with respiratory symptoms. It is cost-effective imaging method and is associated with a very low level of ionizing radiation exposure. We assess the lung aeration, the presence and degree


H. Sago et al. (eds.), *Congenital Cystic Lung Disease*, https://doi.org/10.1007/978-981-15-5175-8_6

of the mediastinal displacement in patients with CCLD from chest radiography, and use it in follow-up.

### 6.2.2 Computed Tomography: CT

The development of multidetector CT (MDCT), which can improve the scan time be short, has increased the role of CT in the assessment of pediatric airways and lungs [1]. In addition, recently introduced high-pitch spiral CT and area-detected CT are helpful in reducing motion artifacts on CT of children with free breathing during the scanning [2]. Therefore, the image quality is further improved by appropriate technologies as follows: a low kilovoltage level for enhanced CT, a high-frequency reconstruction algorithm for lung evaluation, and a standard reconstruction algorism for mediastinal evaluation. CT scan with thinner collimation (less than 1 mm) give us better quality multiplanar reconstruction (MPR) and three-dimensional (3D) images [3].

Although CT is most important modality for diagnosis of CCLD, reduction the CT radiation dose performing diagnostic image quality is of critical importance in pediatric patient, especially neonate, because of the grater radio-sensitivity and longer life expectancy. CT in a single phase of contrast injection is adequate for evaluation of CCLD.

### 6.2.3 Magnetic Resonance Imaging: MRI

Chest MRI has several limitations to assess the lung parenchyma because of the low proton density of the lungs, cardiac and respiratory motion artifact, and susceptibility artifacts that occur at air–tissue interfaces in the lung. Superior tissue contrast resolution and lack of ionizing radiation exposure are big advantages of MRI. Therefore, MRI is nowadays widely used in the pediatric patients with mediastinal mass or chest wall diseases. The development of new technologies of MRI has a possibility to visualize the lung and airway diseases [4, 5].

### 6.2.4 Ultrasound: US

US is another modality which has no radiation exposure. Additionally, it has several advantages in neonates, such as no sedation requirement, real-time observation, wide availability, and portability [6]. Pleural effusion, mediastinal structure, such as large vessels and thymus, are easily evaluated by US. Lung, which contains air, is difficult to visualize on US, while the cystic lesions or consolidations of the lung can assess by US. Color Doppler US is useful to evaluate the abnormal vessels in which the lung lesion suspected bronchopulmonary sequestration [6].

## 6.3 Bronchial Obstruction

### 6.3.1 Congenital Bronchial Atresia

Bronchial atresia (BA) is an anomaly characterized by atresia of a lobar, segmental, or subsegmental bronchus at or near origin, with preservation of the distal bronchus. BAs most frequently affect a segmental bronchus, and most pediatric BAs are congenital. The certain etiology of BA is unknown, but it may be due to a vascular insult in utero [7]. Histologically, the affected bronchus may be obstructed by circumferential or eccentric luminal fibrosis with or without abnormalities of the cartilage and filled with mucin in the bronchi distal to the atretic bronchus create a mucocele [8]. Involvement of multiple segments has been reported [9]. BA is usually diagnosed with incidental findings in older children and adults, or with recurrent pneumonia. Recently, BA diagnosed in antenatal is increased, because of widespread use of prenatal imaging [10].

Segmental overinflation and mucocele are characteristic imaging findings of BA, and CT is the most useful for evaluating these findings

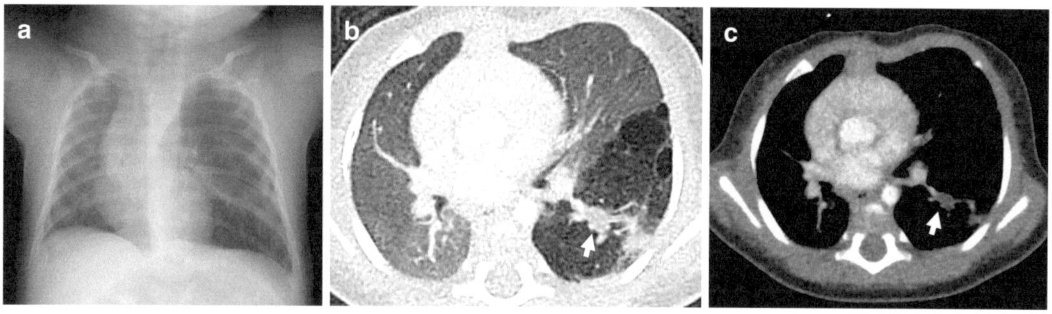


**Fig. 6.1** Bronchial atresia in a 4-month-old with prenatal diagnosis of microcystic type CCLD. (**a**) Frontal chest radiograph shows hyperlucency of the left lower lobe with contralateral mediastinal shift. (**b**) CT image with lung window shows hyperinflation and hyperlucency of the upper segment of left lower lobe due to air-trapping. Segmental bronchus of affected lung is atretic and small bronchial mucocele is shown (arrow). Several small cysts under 5 mm in diameter are demonstrated in the affected segment. (**c**) Bronchial mucocele is demonstrated as a low-density structure on the CT with mediastinal window (arrow)

(Fig. 6.1). Air enters the affected region via collateral ventilation, such as Lambert channel and pole of Kohn, producing air-trapping and hyperinflation [11]. The affected segment may remain atelectasis or consolidation in neonates, because of the delayed lung fluid absorption [12]. Therefore, we should assess carefully in neonate period. Bronchial mucocele is shown in variable size and shape, such as linear, branched, ovoid, or spherical. There are often several cysts containing air in the affected area and they tend to be infection. The cysts may be due to bronchial obstruction, and similar cysts are also found with bronchopulmonary sequestration and type 2 CPAM [7] (Fig. 6.1).

### 6.3.2 Infantile Lobar Emphysema/Congenital Lobar Emphysema

Congenital lobar emphysema (CLE) is characterized by progressive hyperinflation of a lobe, as the result of a partial or complete obstruction of the bronchus by intrinsic or extrinsic factors. The upper lobes are affected more frequently than the lower lobes, with the left lung affected more often than the right [13]. The bronchial narrowing is believed to result in a check-valve mechanism, with progressive hyperinflation of the involved lobe after birth.

CLHs are usually diagnosed by the characteristic radiographic features of progressive lobar overexpansion and hyperlucency, with displacement and compression of adjacent structures such as mediastinum and ipsilateral lobes. Similar imaging findings are shown on CT, which are an expanded hemithorax, an overinflated low-attenuation lobe with stretching the pulmonary vessels, and atelectasis of the adjacent lobes (Fig. 6.2) [ 14]. CT is also useful to evaluate the other causes of lobar emphysema, such as mediastinal mass or vascular anomalies.

## 6.4 Congenital Pulmonary Airway Malformation: CPAM

CPAM, previously known as cystic adenomatoid malformations (CCAM), is developmental anomaly of the lung, that is separated into five types (type 0 to type 4) based on clinical and pathologic features (see also Chap. 14).

Postnatal imaging findings of CPAMs are correlated with underlying pathologic features [14]. On CT imaging, CPAMs are divided into large cyst (larger than 2 cm, type 1, most common), medium or small cyst (less than 2 cm, type 2, 10% to 15%), and solid (microcystic, type 3, very rare). CPAM blood supply is typically from the pulmonary artery and venous drainage is into the pulmonary veins.

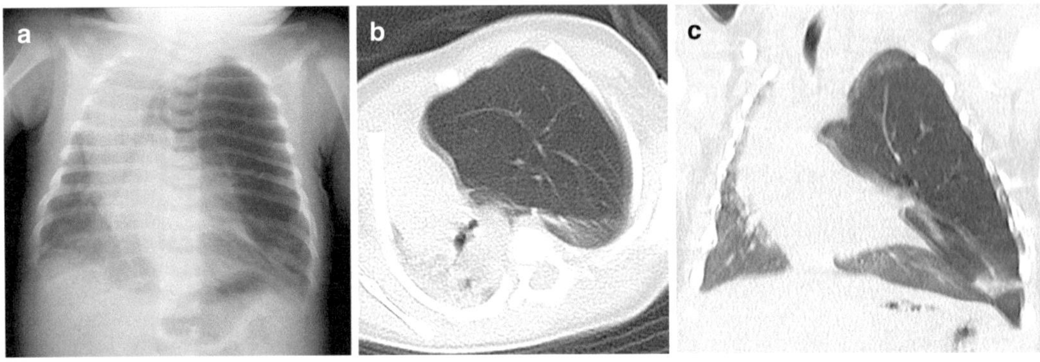


**Fig. 6.2** Congenital lobar emphysema in a 3-week-old with increasing tachypnea. (**a**) Frontal chest radiograph shows hyperexpansion and hyperlucency of the left upper lobe with displacement of mediastinum. (**b**, **c**) CT images demonstrate that overinflated low-attenuation with stretching the pulmonary vessels of the left upper lobe, and atelectasis of the ipsilateral lung

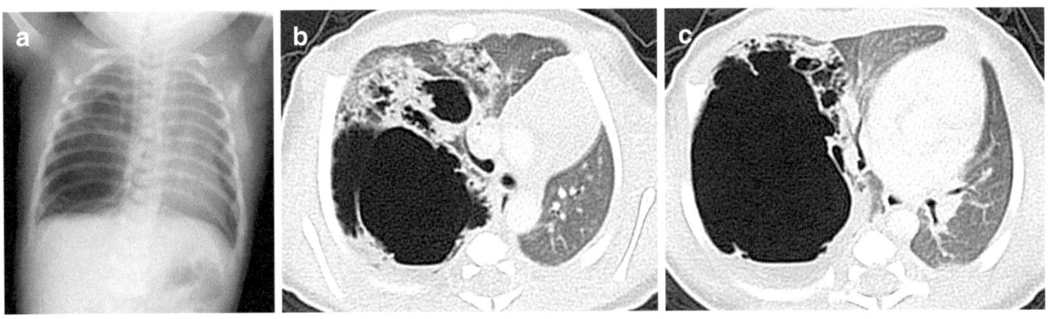


**Fig. 6.3** Congenital pulmonary airway malformation type 1 in a 4-day-old neonate with prenatal diagnosis of macrocystic CCLD. (**a**) Frontal chest radiograph shows large hyperlucent area with displacement to mediastinum and adjacent lobe of the right lung. (**b**, **c**) CT images with lung window show a large cystic mass containing air and fluid with thick wall with contralateral mediastinal shift. Multiple several sized cysts are shown surrounding the large cyst

The type 1 lesions are characterized by single or multiple large cysts (2 to 10 cm in diameter) surrounded by smaller cysts and compressed normal parenchyma (Fig. 6.3). The wall of large cyst is often thick and irregular. CPAMs with significant mediastinal shift lead to respiratory symptom, and need surgical intervention, such as lobectomy, in early life of a patient.

The type 2 lesions are composed of cyst 0.5 to 2 cm in diameter. Type 2 CPAMs are sometimes found because of a pneumonia or a lung abscess, which are similar with intralobar sequestration or BA with multiple cysts both on clinically and radiologically.

The type 3 CPAMs consist of a large, bulky, parenchymal mass involving an entire lobe or even an entire lung. Because type 3 cysts are very small (rarely larger than 0.2 cm in diameter), the lesions of type 3 are typically shown as solid mass with mild contrast enhancement on CT or MRI. The cases of type 3 are frequently associated with other anomalies and have a high mortality.

The lesion of type 4 CPAM (15%) appears as a large cyst at the periphery of the lung and may be difficult to distinguish radiologically from cystic pleuropulmonary blastoma. Recently, type 4 CPAMs are proposed to the same entity as type 1 (pure cystic type) pleuropulmonary blastoma [15].

## 6.5 Bronchopulmonary Sequestration: BPS

BPS is defined as a congenital lung malformation disconnected from normal bronchial tree with its systemic arterial supply, characteristic by combined parenchymal and vascular lesions of the lung [16]. Systemic arterial supply is usually from aorta, and it may arise from branches of the celiac, intercostal, or subclavian artery. The presence of abnormal systemic vessels is important to diagnose the sequestration, and color Doppler US, contrast-enhanced CT, and MRI are modality to demonstrate the vessels (Figs. 6.4 and 6.5). Multidetector CT with contrast medium is considered the imaging technique of choice for preoperative evaluation of pulmonary sequestration [3, 17]. Multiplanar and 3D-CT images have the advantage of being able to show the pulmonary parenchymal abnormality, as well as the arterial and venous architecture of the sequestration.

BPS is divided into two groups: extralobar (25%) and intralobar (75%), and intralobar sequestration (ILS) is located within the left lower lobe in 60% of the cases. The cases in the upper lobe and in the middle lobe are rare.

Extralobar sequestrations (ELSs) are discrete masses of pulmonary parenchyma outside the normal pleural. On chest radiograph, ELS typically presents as a focal nonaerated mass, usually located between the lower lobe and diaphragm (Fig. 6.4). On CT and MRI, ELSs characteristi-

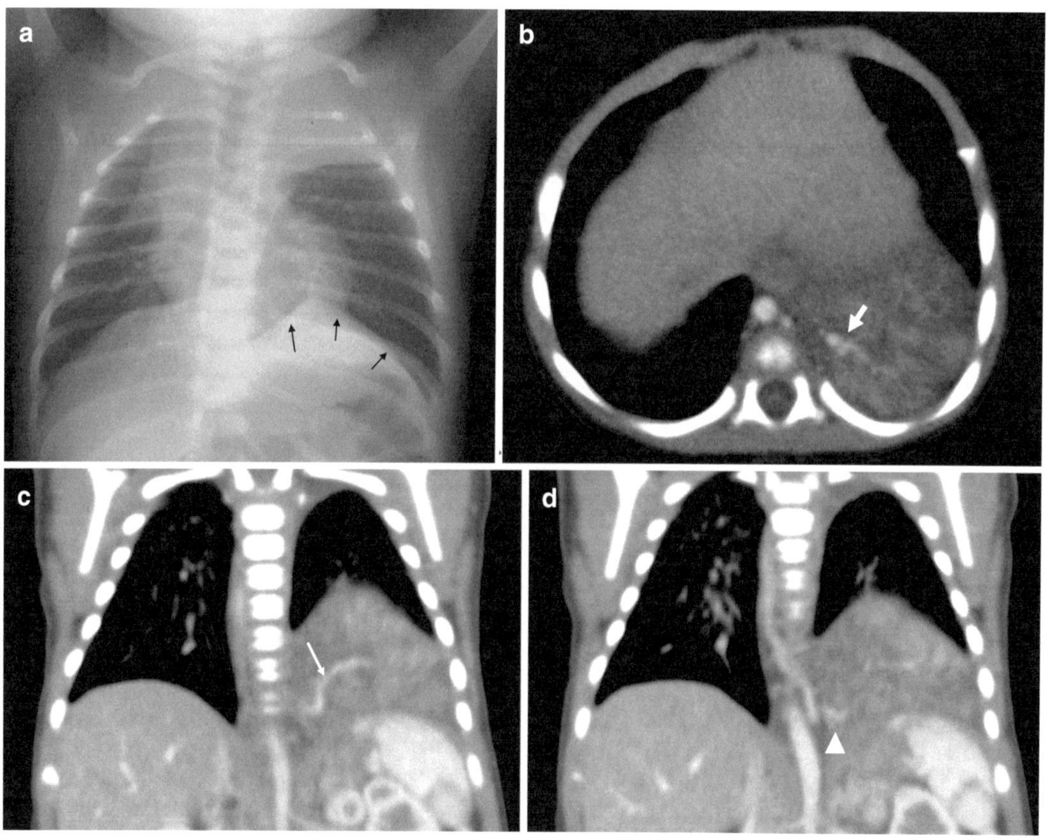


**Fig. 6.4** Extralobar sequestration in a 2-week-old with no respiratory symptom. (**a**) Frontal chest radiograph shows tent-like shadow in the left pulmonary base (arrows). (**b**) Contrast-enhanced CT shows the mass with heterogeneous enhancement of the left lung base and a systemic branching vessel originating from the aorta (arrow). (**c**, **d**) Coronal multiplanar reconstruction CT images show unaerated, enhancing mass-like lesion in the left lung base with arteries from the aorta (arrow) and vessels draining to the azygos vein (arrow head). Mass-like lesion is separated from normal lung tissue with sharp and clarified margin suggested extrapulmonary location

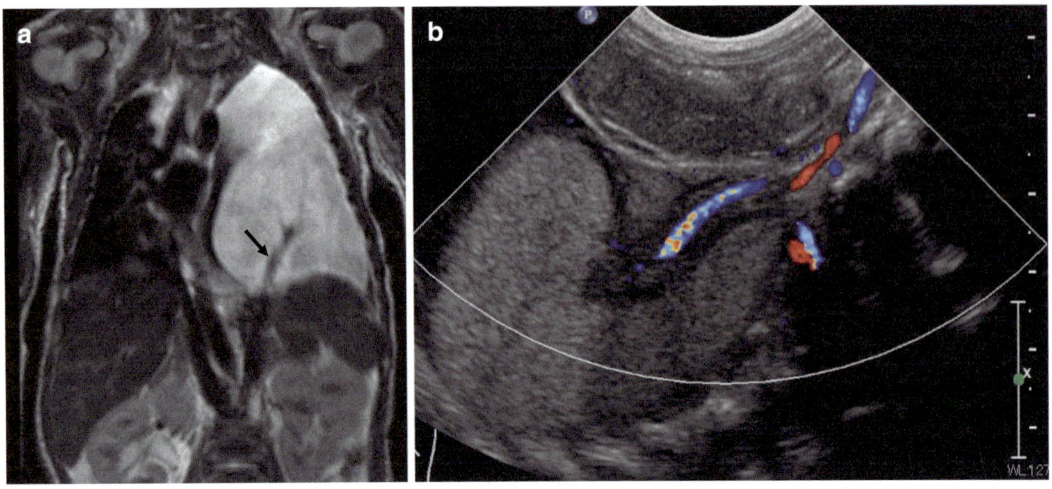


**Fig. 6.5** Extralobar sequestration in a 1-day-old neonate. (**a**) Coronal T2-weighted MR image shows a large high signal intensity mass in the left hemithorax with a flow void (arrow) which suggested abnormal systemic vessels from abdominal aorta. (**b**) Transverse Color Doppler shows the abnormal vessels originating at the aorta and supplying the mass

cally are shown as solid, unaerated mass lesions, and vascular supply occurs through a systemic artery and venous drainage through the azygos or portal vein (Fig. 6.4), although nearly 25% are completely or partially drained by pulmonary vein. Most cases of ELS are asymptomatic and ELS may show spontaneous regression during pregnancy and infancy [18]. ELSs are rarely infected because of no communication with bronchial tree, and ESLs with hemorrhagic necrosis due to torsion in childhood have been reported [19].

Intralobar sequestration (ILS) consists of a portion of lung within the normal pleural investment that is isolated/sequestered from the tracheobronchial tree and is supplied by systemic artery, typically embedded within a normal lobe. On chest radiograph, ILSs often present as a focal lung mass and/or cyst but also may be shown as a consolidation of the lung (Fig. 6.6).

On CT, ILS lesions are shown as unaerated area or consolidation in the normal lung, with and without cysts, because the lesions are not separated by the pleura. ILSs may be found several small cysts, similar findings of BA and type 2 CPAM, and may present hyperlucent area due to air-trapping [7] (Fig. 6.6). Anomalous vascular components of ILS can be evaluated with CT or MRI, same as ELS, but it may be difficult to prove the anomalous vessels because of inflammatory changes with superimposed infection.

## 6.6 Foregut Duplication Cysts

Foregut duplication cysts result from abnormal budding of the tracheal diverticulum, including of bronchogenic cysts, enteric duplication cysts and foregut cysts, usually are located within the mediastinum. These cysts are seen most frequently as incidental findings, but may present with symptoms related to secondary infection of the cyst.

Bronchogenic cysts are most frequent in the mediastinum, predominantly near the carina, it may be located anywhere from suprasternal area to the retroperitoneum [20]. It also may be found in the lung parenchyma, usually in the lower lobe. Bronchogenic cysts typically are unilocular, fluid-filled or mucin-filled cysts and are attached to, but rarely connected to, the tracheobronchial tree.

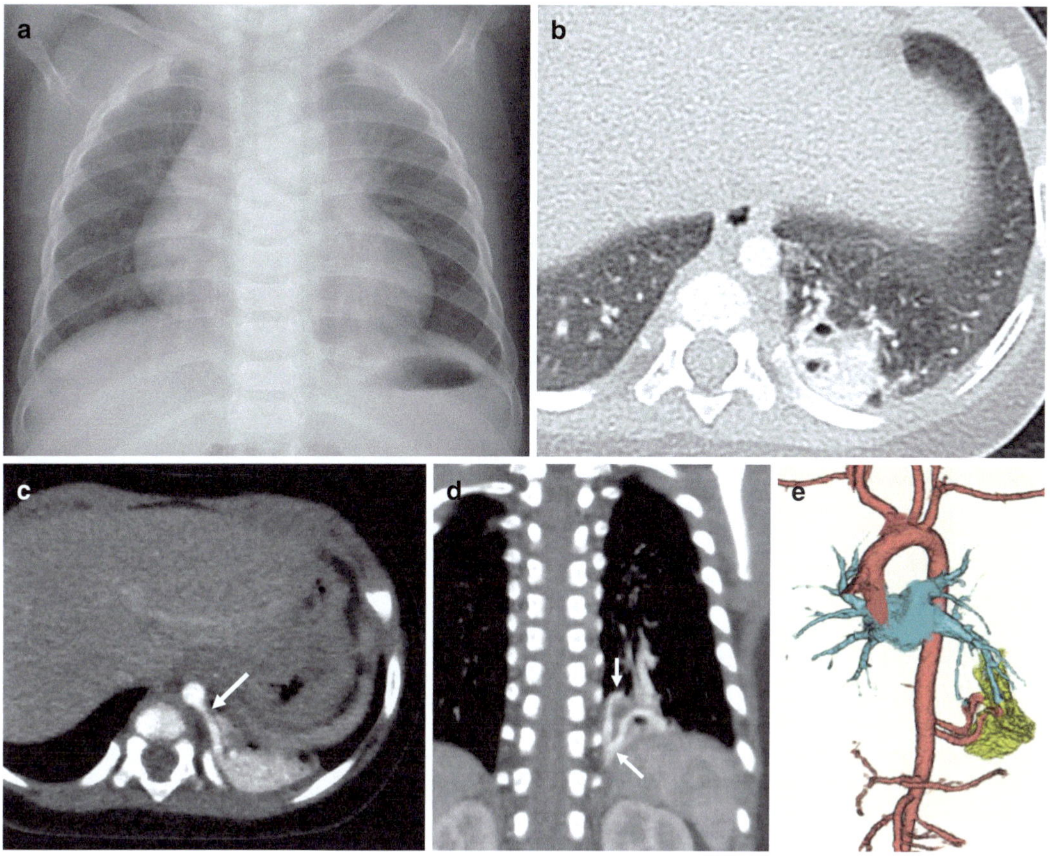

**Fig. 6.6** Intralobar sequestration with prenatal diagnosis of microcystic CCLD. (**a**) Frontal chest radiograph shows small consolidation in the left lower lobe. (**b**, **c**) Contrast-enhanced CT images demonstrate unaerated area with a systemic vessel (arrow) in the left lower lobe. Small air-containing cysts and hyperlucent area around consolidation are shown. These are suggested the presence of airway obstruction. (**d**, **e**) Coronal multiplanar reconstruction CT image and 3D-CT demonstrate two vessels from the aorta to sequestration (arrows)

On chest radiograph, a cyst manifests as a well-delineated round or oval-shaped mediastinal mass. US, CT, and MR allow a better evaluation of cysts and its anatomic relationship with adjacent structure. US and MRI are better than CT to evaluate for differentiating a cyst from a solid mass without contrast medium, there is also the advantage that there is no radiation exposure. On MRI, cysts are homogeneously and markedly high signal intensity on T2-weighted images and the wall of the cyst is thin (Fig. 6.7). The intra-cystic signal intensity on T1-weighted images is variable, depending upon the cyst content [21]. Relatively high signal intensity on T1-weighted images is due to a high protein content and or the bleeding. The presence of an air-fluid level, thick wall of the cyst (may be with enhancement) is suggested for superimposed infection [12].

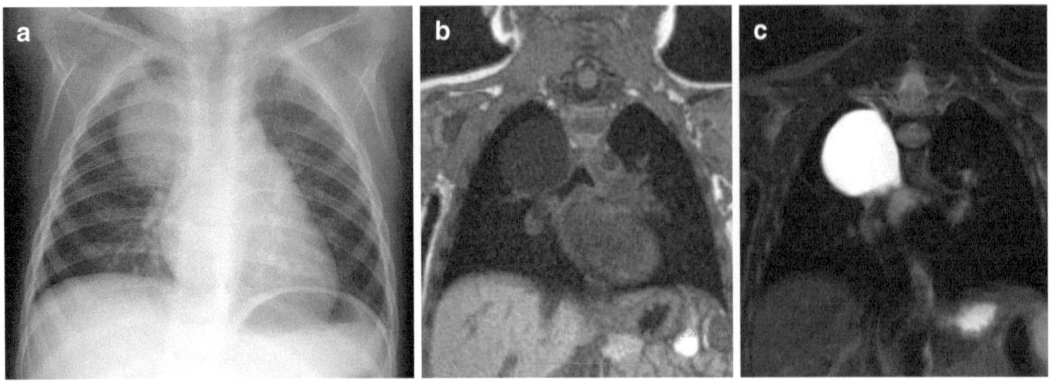


**Fig. 6.7** Mediastinal bronchogenic cyst in 3-year-old boy. (**a**) Frontal chest radiograph shows a spherical right mediastinal mass. (**b**) Coronal T1-weighted MR image demonstrates the presence of a low signal intensity mass of right perihilar region. (**c**) The mass is shown very high signal intensity on coronal T2-weighted MR image

## References

1. Lemos AA, Siegel MJ, Rossi G, et al. Single-versus multidetector-row CT: comparison of sedation rates, conventional angiograms and motion artefacts in young children following liver transplantation. Radiol Med. 2006 Oct;111(7):911–20.
2. Lell MM, May M, Deak P, et al. High-pitch spiral computed tomography: effect on image quality and radiation dose in pediatric chest computed tomography. Investig Radiol. 2011 Feb;46(2):116–23.
3. Siegel MJ. Multiplanar and three-dimensional multi-detector row CT of thoracic vessels and airways in the pediatric population. Radiology. 2003 Dec;229(3):641–50.
4. Niwa T, Nozawa K, Aida N. Visualization of the airway in infants with MRI using pointwise encoding time reduction with radial acquisition (PETRA). J Magn Reson Imaging. 2017 Mar;45(3):839–44.
5. Dournes G, Grodzki D, Macey J, et al. Quiet submillimeter MR imaging of the lung is feasible with a PETRA sequence at 1.5 T. Radiology. 2016 Apr;279(1):328.
6. Coley BD. Chest sonography in children: current indications, techniques, andimaging findings. Radiol Clin N Am. 2011 Sep;49(5):825–46.
7. Langston C. New concepts in the pathology of congenital lung malformations. Semin Pediatr Surg. 2003 Feb;12(1):17–37.
8. Lemire P, Trepanier A, Hebert G. Bronchocele and blocked bronchiectasis. Am J Roentgenol. 1970;110:687–93.
9. Ward S, Morcos SK. Congenital bronchial atresia. Presentation of three cases and a pictorial review. Clin Radiol. 1999;54:144–8.
10. Riedlinger WF, Vargas SO, Jennings RW, et al. Bronchial atresia is common to extralobar sequestration, intralobar sequestration, congenital cystic adenomatoid malformation, and lobar emphysema. Pediatr Dev Pathol. 2006 Sep-Oct;9(5):361–73.
11. Talner LB, Gmelich JT, Liebow AA, et al. The syndrome of bronchial mucocele and regional hyperinflation of the lung. Am J Roentgenol Radium Therapy, Nucl Med. 1970 Dec;110(4):675–86.
12. Epelman M, Kreiger PA, Servaes S, et al. Current imaging of prenatally diagnosed congenital lung lesions. Semin Ultrasound CT MR. 2010 Apr;31(2):141–57.
13. Mani H, Suarez E, Stocker JT. The morphologic spectrum of infantile lobar emphysema: a study of 33 cases. Paediatr Respir Rev. 2004;5:S313–20.
14. Biyyam DR, Chapman T, Ferguson MR, et al. Congenital lung abnormalities: embryologic features, prenatal diagnosis, and postnatal radiologic-pathologic correlation. Radiographics. 2010 Oct;30(6):1721–38.
15. Priest JR, Williams GM, Hill DA, et al. Pulmonary cysts in early childhood and the risk of malignancy. Pediatr Pulmonol. 2009 Jan;44(1):14–30.
16. Heitzman ER. The lung: radiologic-pathologic correlations. St Louis: Mosby; 1984.
17. Lee EY, Siegel MJ, Sierra LM, et al. Evaluation of angioarchitecture of pulmonary sequestration in pediatric patients using 3D MDCT angiography. Am J Roentgenol. 2004;183:183–8.
18. Yoon HM, Kim EA, Chung SH, et al. Extralobar pulmonary sequestration in neonates: the natural course and predictive factors associated with spontaneous regression. Eur Radiol. 2017 Jun;27(6):2489–96.
19. Chen W, Wagner L, Boyd T, Nagarajan R, Dasgupta R. Extralobar pulmonary sequestration presenting with torsion: a case report and review of literature. J Pediatr Surg. 2011 Oct;46(10):2025–8.
20. McAdams HP, Kirejczyk WM, Rosaro-Christenson ML, et al. Bronchogenic cyst: imaging features with clinical and histopathologic correlation. Radiology. 2000;217:441–6.
21. Lyon RD, McAdams HP. Mediastinal bronchogenic cyst demonstration of a fluid-fluid level at MR imaging. Radiology. 1993;186:427–8.

# 7 Perinatal Natural History and Treatment of Congenital Lung Malformations in Prenatally Diagnosed Neonates

Toshihiko Watanabe

**Abstract**

Congenital lung malformations comprise a spectrum of disease entities, including congenital pulmonary airway malformation, bronchial atresia, and intra- and extralobar sequestration. With the progress in prenatal diagnosis, fetuses diagnosed as CLM has been increasing. However, the perinatal clinical features of each disease have not yet been described. They comprise a broad spectrum of symptom ranging from complete regression of the lesion to rapid growth resulting in hydrops fetalis. In addition, the indication and the timing for surgery are still controversial. Thus, strategy to evaluate patients' degree of severity and customize treatment to each patient's particular need is vital. We have three types of surgical timings; standby emergency surgery for respiratory failure just after planned cesarean section, emergency surgery for respiratory distress in neonatal period and elective surgery for asymptomatic children around 1 year of age. The prognosis is quite excellent in non-hydrotropic fetuses. The outcome is still poor in spite of planned fetal interventions and standby emergency surgery in neonates with hydrops fetalis. The alternative strategy is needed for the better outcome of these severer hydrotropic fetuses.

**Keywords**

Congenital lung malformation · Congenital pulmonary airway malformation · Congenital cystic adenomatoid malformation · Bronchial atresia · Prenatal diagnosis · Children

## 7.1 Introduction

Congenital lung malformations (CLM) are rare and diverse in their presentation. Understanding the pathophysiology of these malformations is important because potential consequences can be life threatening. CLM represents a spectrum of developmental conditions, including congenital pulmonary airway malformation (CPAM), bronchopulmonary sequestration, bronchogenic cyst, congenital lobar emphysema, and bronchial atresia (BA) [1, 2]. Definitive diagnosis can be identified by distinct pathological findings after surgery; therefore, we have to manage fetus or infants according to their clinical conditions. In this section, perinatal clinical features of congenital cystic lung disease with a focus on the definitive diagnosis will be discussed.

T. Watanabe (✉)
Department of Pediatric Surgery, Tokai University School of Medicine, Kanagawa, Isehara, Japan

Division of Surgery, National Center for Child Health and Development, Tokyo, Japan
e-mail: watanabe-ts@tsc.u-tokai.ac.jp



H. Sago et al. (eds.), *Congenital Cystic Lung Disease*, https://doi.org/10.1007/978-981-15-5175-8_7

## 7.2 Diversity in Congenital Lung Malformations

The nomenclature of CLM has been confusing because of rarity of these lesions estimated at 1 per 20,000 to 30,000 live birth [3] resulting in insufficient evidence base. Several factors associated with these lesions including timing of diagnosis (prenatally or postnatally), morphologies (solid or cystic), condition (symptomatic or asymptomatic), and considerable overlap of histologic features within the same lesion ("hybrid" lesion) [4] make this issue more ambiguous. The condition of the patient generally depends on the size of the affected pulmonary lobe caused by compression on surrounding organs [3, 4]. Bronchogenic cyst, extralobar sequestration, lobar emphysema, and CPAM are often assumed to be separate identities and have distinct pathological features [2, 5]. Awareness of fetal diagnosis of CLM has been increasing by obstetricians. In our center, cases with fetal diagnosis have exceeded non-fetal diagnosis from 2008. Yearly trend regarding percentage of prenatally diagnosed patients revealed the gradual increase up to 100% during the last 15 years (Fig. 7.1).

## 7.3 Bronchial Atresia as a Distinct Entity

Since Shuster et al. reported BA as a recognizable disease entity in 1978 [6], there has been debate for decades if BA is one component of a number of different congenital lung abnormalities [4, 7–10] or distinct entity [6, 11–13]. Diagnosis of BA was made by gross morphological analysis and histological findings of a blind-ending bronchus associated with a distal mucous filled bronchocele surrounded by hyperinflated or cystic structured lung parenchyma. Typical microscopic features of CPAM included bronchus-like structures with muscle, glands, and cartilage plates, or pseudostratified columnar epithelial lining of the cyst. We investigated 112 patients who were diagnosed pathologically as CPAM or BA in an attempt to clarify the characteristics of BA in infants and children and to describe the spectrum of this condition [14]. Seventy-one patients were diagnosed prenatally and 41 postnatally. Percentage of prenatal diagnosis was significantly higher in CPAM patients (84% vs 50%, $p < 0.001$). Among patients with prenatal diagnosis, the backgrounds were not different between the two diseases except the

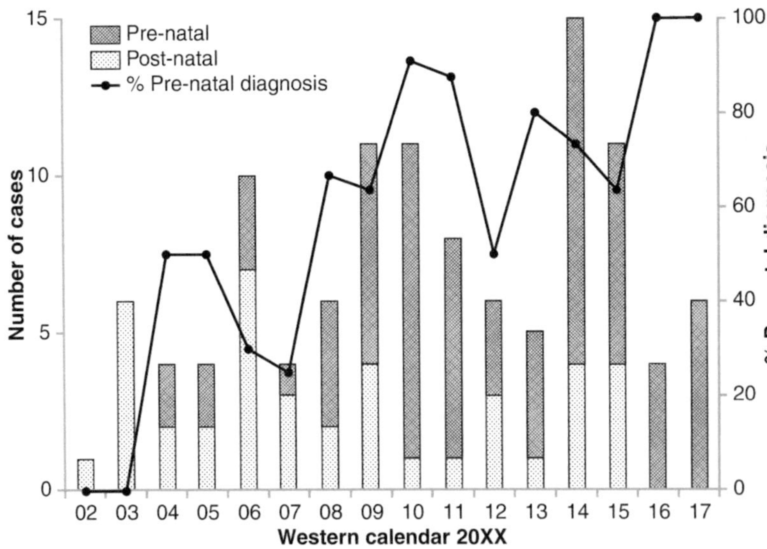


**Fig. 7.1** Yearly trend on percentage of prenatally diagnosed patients

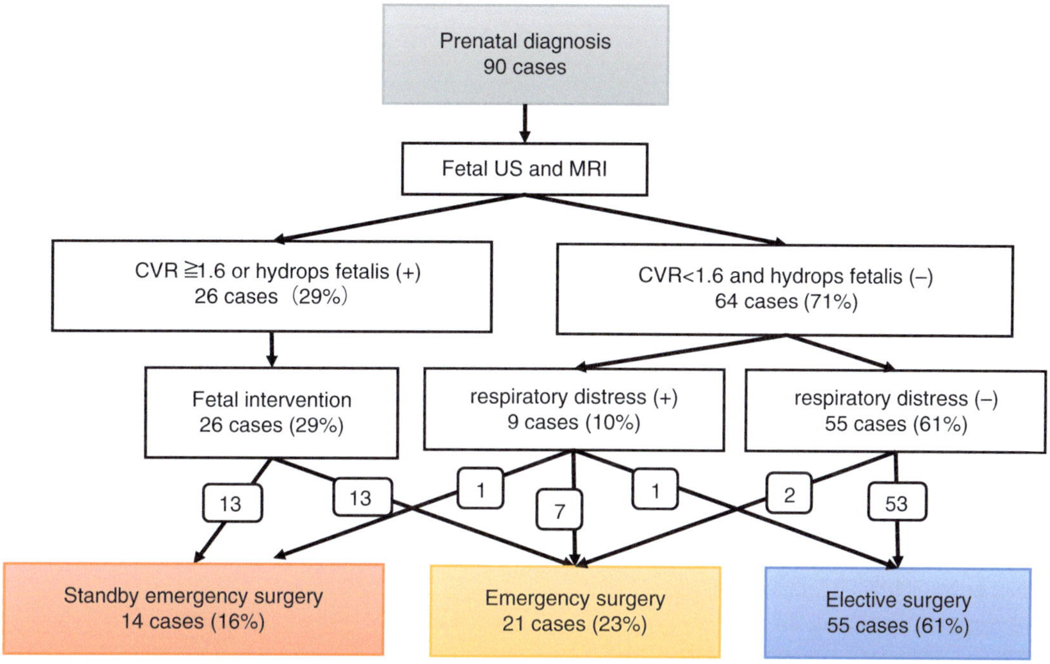


**Fig. 7.2** Flowchart of treatment in prenatally diagnosed patients

number of Caesarean section (81% vs 9%, $p < 0.0001$). The numbers of patients that underwent fetal interventions and emergent neonatal surgery were higher in CPAM (51% vs 15%, $p < 0.01$, 76% vs 12%, $p < 0.0001$), although there was no statistical difference in survival rate (86% vs 97%, $p = 0.2$). In patients diagnosed postnatally, pneumonia was the primary symptom in most of BA patients, whereas respiratory distress was the major symptom in patients with CPAM. Age at developing the primary symptom was significantly older in BA patients (4.2 y vs 1.2 y, $p < 0.005$). Thus, CPAM and BA have distinct clinical features in terms of therapeutic and natural history. There is a need for individual therapeutic algorithm.

## 7.4 Postnatal Natural History, Treatment, and Prognosis

CLM with prenatal diagnosis has been gradually increasing in recent years. Therefore, strategy of the treatment policy after birth based on degree of fetal severity has become important. For the 15-year study period, 90 patients with prenatal diagnosis were experienced pulmonary resection due to CLM. Our flowchart of treatment option depending on severity of fetal disease is shown in Fig. 7.2. Fetal lung mass are assessed by ultrasonography and MRI. In fetuses with CCAM volume ratio (CVR) ≧ 1.6 or hydrops fetalis, fetal interventions such as shunt placement for macrocystic cysts or maternal steroid administration for microcystic cysts are considered. These fetuses account for 29% of the fetuses with prenatal diagnosis. There are three types of surgical timing. Standby emergency surgery is carried out in fetuses with severe disease taking into account the risk of respiratory failure immediately after birth. Anesthesiologist, neonatologist, and surgeon are on standby for resuscitation and operation in the next room of maternal cesarean section (Fig. 7.3). Emergency surgery is conducted when respiratory distress is seen in neonates in NICU. Sixteen-one percent of the patients are asymptomatic and experience surgery electively. Enhanced CT, bronchoscopy, bronchography, and angiography were examined for asymptomatic patients around 8–10 month-old

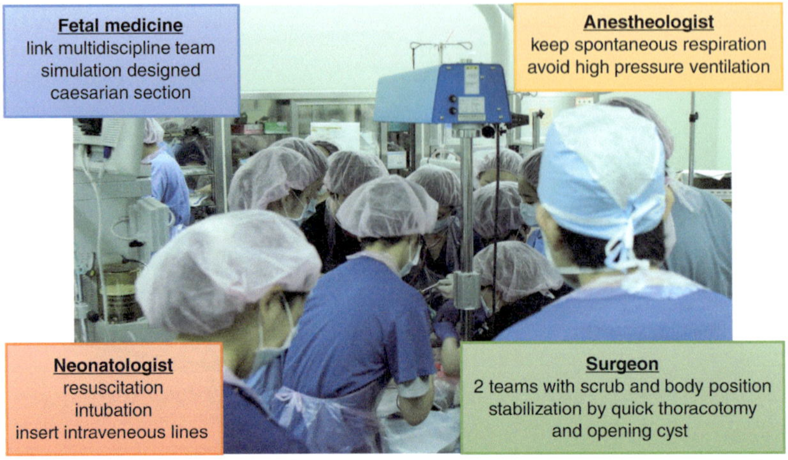


**Fig. 7.3** Standby emergency surgery

under general anesthesia. Radiological images of bronchography and angiography were compared whether bronchial atresia exists or not, and tentative clinical diagnosis was made. Elective surgery was projected thereafter around 1 year of age regardless of clinical diagnosis.

Surgical outcome is shown in Table 7.1. Standby emergency surgery is planned in 16% of the neonates and the median time of operation after birth was 40 minutes with a range from 14 to 108 minutes. Three cases died with survival rate of 79%. Emergency surgery was performed in 22% of the cases with a survival rate of 75%. Elective surgery was performed in 62% of the patients at a median of 416 days without death.

The breakdown for each surgical timing is unique and significant to understand behavior of each disease entity on CLM after birth (Fig. 7.4). All neonates who required standby emergency surgery are pathologically diagnosed as CPAM type I. CPAM is still the major disease entity (67%) which have respiratory distress in NICU resulting in emergency surgery. Meanwhile, BA is the major disease for elective surgery. CCAM is likely to discover in prenatal period. Some patients have poor prognosis despite fetal intervention and neonatal emergency surgery. BA and ILS have good prognosis with stable prenatal period and less morbidity of respiratory distress after birth [15].

Figure 7.5 shows an example case with standby emergency surgery. This baby was born at 2435 g with 38th gestational weeks. He cried very weakly several times, but then stopped spontaneous breathing. Chest X-ray revealed extreme midline shift (A). Since heart rate became less than 60 per minutes, neonatologist started adrenaline administration and sternum compression for about 3 minutes. HFO respira-

**Table. 7.1** Outcome by timing of operation

| | Standby emergency surgery ($n$=14) | Emergency surgery ($n$=21) | Elective surgery ($n$=55) |
|---|---|---|---|
| GA at diagnosis | 21 (18–31) | 23 (17–30) | 23 (14–56) |
| Hydrops fetalis | 50% | 38% | 0% |
| Fetal intervention | 93% | 57% | 2% |
| GA at delivery | 37 (28–39) | 38 (35–39) | 38 (35–39) |
| Birth weight(g) | 2789 (1490–4070) | 2862 (1852–3500) | 2956 (1828–3613) |
| APGAR 1(min) | 7 (1–8) | 8 (1–8) | 8 (4–9) |
| APGAR 5(min) | 8 (1–9) | 9 (2–9) | 9 (4–10) |
| Timing of surgery | 40 (14–108) (min) | 1 (0-30) (day) | 416 (51–1586) (day) |
| Operation time(min) | 94.5 (36–161) | 112 (57–192) | 177 (55–481) |
| Deceased case | 3 cases | 4 cases | none |
| Survival rate | 79% | 81% | 100% |

**Fig. 7.4** Pathological diagnosis by timing of operation

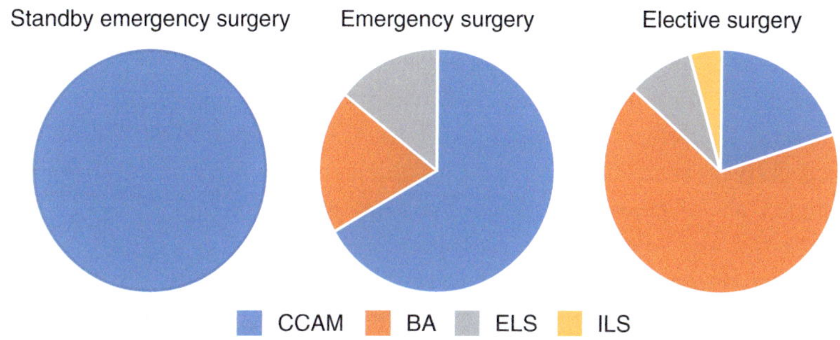


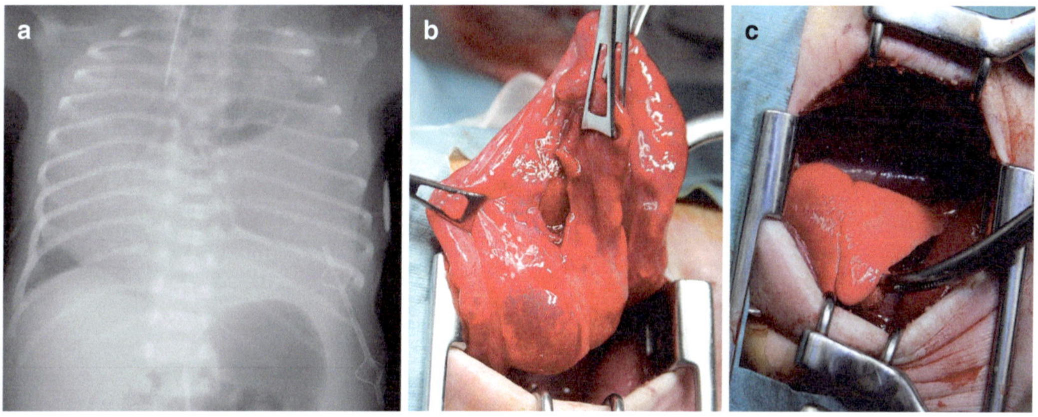


**Fig. 7.5** An example case with standby emergency surgery

**Table. 7.2** Demographics of deceased cases

| Gestational week | Birth weight(g) | Hydrops fetalis | CVR | Fetal intervention | Timing of surgery | Pathological diagnosis |
|---|---|---|---|---|---|---|
| 35 | 2810 | (+) | 2.3 | (+) | Standby emergency | CCAM type I |
| 28 | 1490 | (+) | 5.4 | (+) | Standby emergency | CCAM type I |
| 36 | 2950 | (+) | 3.9 | (+) | Standby emergency | CCAM type I |
| 28 | 1852 | (+) | 5.5 | (+) | Emergency | Extralobar sequestration |
| 36 | 3500 | (+) | 2.0 | (+) | Emergency | CCAM type I |
| 35 | 2224 | (+) | 3.0 | (+) | Emergency | BA |
| 34 | 3152 | (+) | 5.0 | (+) | Emergency | CCAM type I |

tory management, securing the blood vessel line of the arteriovenous, surgery started in 17 minutes after birth. A huge cyst was opened and brought out of the thoracic cavity, resulting in stabilization of circulation at 21 minutes after birth (B). Lower left lobe was removed in 1 hour 37 minutes (C). Histopathological examination was CCAM type I. Planned standby emergency surgery and multidisciplinary team overcame this life-threatening condition.

Demographics of six deceased cases is shown in Table 7.2. Premature infants, developing hydrops fetalis and high CVR over 2.0 are high risk parameters for neonatal demise after surgery. All patients received fetal interventions and emergency surgery. Pathological diagnosis was three cases for CCAM type I; two cases for type III; and one for ELS. Once fetus develops hydrops fetalis, the survival rate was extremely poor at 50%.

Establishing the algorithm of management for prenatally diagnosed lung disease and sharing the fetal information across all relevant departments are vital. Definitive criterion for fetal intervention and delivery plan including standby emergency surgery are of great importance. The fetus with large cyst can be rescued by combining standby emergency surgery with fetal intervention. The prognosis is quite excellent in non-hydrotropic fetuses. The outcome is still poor in spite of planned fetal interventions and standby emergency surgery in neonates with hydrops fetalis. The alternative strategy is needed for the better outcome of these severer hydrotropic fetuses.

## References


1. Stocker JT. Cystic lung disease in infants and children. Fetal Pediatr Pathol. 2009;28:155–84.
2. Langston C. New concepts in the pathology of congenital lung malformations. Semin Pediatr Surg. 2003;12:17–37.
3. Laberge JM, Flageole H, Pugash D, Khalife S, Blair G, Filiatrault D, Russo P, Lees G, Wilson RD. Outcome of the prenatally diagnosed congenital cystic adenomatoid lung malformation: a Canadian experience. Fetal Diagn Ther. 2001;16:178–86.
4. Cass DL, Crombleholme TM, Howell LJ, Stafford PW, Ruchelli ED, Adzick NS. Cystic lung lesions with systemic arterial blood supply: a hybrid of congenital cystic adenomatoid malformation and bronchopulmonary sequestration. J Pediatr Surg. 1997;32:986–90.
5. Fowler DJ, Gould SJ. The pathology of congenital lung lesions. Semin Pediatr Surg. 2015;24:176–82.
6. Schuster SR, Harris GB, Williams A, Kirkpatrick J, Reid L. Bronchial atresia: a recognizable entity in the pediatric age group. J Pediatr Surg. 1978;13:682–9.
7. Disciosclo V, Feraco P, Bazzocchi A, Femia R, Romeo C, Fasano L, Pacilli AM, Zompatori M. Congenital cystic adenomatoid malformation of the lung associated with bronchial atresia involving a different lobe in an adult patient: a case report. J Med Case Rep. 2010;4:164.
8. Kunisaki SM, Fauza DO, Nemes LP, Barnewolt CE, Estroff JA, Kozakewich HP, Jennings RW. Bronchial atresia: the hidden pathology within a spectrum of prenatally diagnosed lung masses. J Pediatr Surg. 2006;41:61–5. Discussion–5
9. Wong KS, Wang CR, Lien R. Bronchial atresia with mucocele in an adolescent girl: an uncommon cause of lobar emphysema. Monaldi Arch Chest Dis. 2000;55:375–7.
10. Riedlinger WF, Vargas SO, Jennings RW, Estroff JA, Barnewolt CE, Lillehei CW, Wilson JM, Colin AA, Reid LM, Kozakewich HP. Bronchial atresia is common to extralobar sequestration, intralobar sequestration, congenital cystic adenomatoid malformation, and lobar emphysema. Pediatr Dev Pathol. 2006;9:361–73.
11. Pedicelli G, Ciarpaglini LL, De Santis M, Leonetti C. Congenital bronchial atresia (CBA). A critical review of CBA as a disease entity and presentation of a case series. Radiol Med. 2005;110:544–53.
12. Morikawa N, Kuroda T, Honna T, Kitano Y, Fuchimoto Y, Terawaki K, Kawasaki K, Koinuma G, Matsuoka K, Saeki M. Congenital bronchial atresia in infants and children. J Pediatr Surg. 2005;40:1822–6.
13. Matsushima H, Takayanagi N, Satoh M, Kurashima K, Kanauchi T, Hoshi T, Kanazawa M. Congenital bronchial atresia: radiologic findings in nine patients. J Comput Assist Tomogr. 2002;26:860–4.
14. Watanabe T, Ohno M, Tahara K, Tomonaga K, Fuchimoto Y, Fujino A, Hishiki T, Tsukamoto K, Ito Y, Sugibayashi R, Wada S, Sago H, Higuchi M, Kawasaki K, Yoshioka T, Kanamori Y. An investigation on clinical differences between congenital pulmonary airway malformation and bronchial atresia. J Pediatr Surg. 2018;53:2390–3.
15. Fuchimoto Y, Watanabe T, Fujino A, Kanamori Y, Itoh Y, Wada S, Sago H, Yoshioka T. Predictors of early lobectomy after birth in prenatally diagnosed congenital pulmonary airway malformation. J Pediatr Surg. 2018;53:2386–9.

# Surgical Treatment for and Prognosis of Congenital Pulmonary Airway Malformation

8

Noriaki Usui

**Abstract**

Congenital pulmonary airway malformation (CPAM) is a congenital disease in which cystic lesions form within the pulmonary parenchyma, because the development of the airway or lung are partially interrupted in the fetal lung development. When considering the indications, timing, procedure, and other aspects of surgery for CPAM, it is imperative to appropriately understand the anatomical and pathophysiological differences between CPAM and other congenital cystic lung diseases (CCLD). The major anatomical characteristic of CPAM is that the cystic lesions are communicated with the normal airways. Since lesions seen in the fetuses with CPAM are generally larger compared with other CCLDs, neonates with CPAM tend to be associated with hydrops and pulmonary hypoplasia and often develop persistent pulmonary hypertension of the newborn (PPHN). Therefore, infants with CPAM have a high risk of severe postnatal respiratory impairment. Surgical treatment during the neonatal period is necessary for the infants with CPAM who reveal any respiratory symptoms after birth. Surgery should be considered even in the asymptomatic cases of CPAM after birth in order to prevent respiratory infection. If all cystic lesions of the CPAM are not treated, the residual cysts could act as a nidus for postoperative infection. Therefore, all affected lesions must be completely resected if the affected lesions are limited in a single lobe. although the affected lesions should be resected as much as possible even in a case of multiple lobes are involved, resection of multiple lobes including total pneumonectomy in a single procedure should be avoided in order to preserve pulmonary functions of the residual lungs.

**Keywords**

Congenital cystic lung disease · Congenital cystic adenomatoid malformation · Congenital pulmonary airway malformation · Stocker's classification · Pulmonary hypoplasia · Persistent pulmonary hypertension of the newborn

## 8.1 Introduction

In recent years, many of the cases of congenital pulmonary airway malformation (CPAM) have been diagnosed prenatally. Some critical cases with a prenatal diagnosis of CPAM may have severe pulmonary hypoplasia that will result in respiratory distress subsequent to birth; meanwhile, other mild cases with a prenatal diagnosis of

N. Usui (✉)
Department of Pediatric Surgery, Osaka Women's and Children's Hospital, Murodo-cho-840, Izumi, Osaka, Japan
e-mail: usui@wch.opho.jp





H. Sago et al. (eds.), *Congenital Cystic Lung Disease*, https://doi.org/10.1007/978-981-15-5175-8_8

CPAM are asymptomatic at birth, and sometimes the lesions of CPAM may even decrease in size afterward [1–3]. In some cases, without a prenatal diagnosis, the symptoms are identified postnatally when the patient develops signs of an infection. Since CPAM involves such a wide range of severities and pathophysiologies, a better understanding of an individual patient's condition and making appropriate decisions are essential for the surgical treatment of the patients with CPAM. This chapter describes the key point of surgical treatment and the prognosis of the patients with CPAM.

## 8.2 Definition

CPAM is a congenital disease in which cystic lesions form within the pulmonary parenchyma, because the development of the fetal airway or lung are partially interrupted due to an abnormal airway pattern occurring during fetal lung branching morphogenesis [4]. CPAM is classified into several types based on the size of the cysts and the area and stage of the developmental interruption in the airway or lung.

## 8.3 Classification

The Stocker's classification of CPAM has been widely used in recent years. In 1977, Stocker had named the condition in which adenomatoid cysts formed from partially interrupted development of the lung or airway as "congenital cystic adenomatoid malformation (CCAM)" [5], and this was used for many years before being renamed as CPAM. Initially, Stocker had classified CCAM into three types based on the similarity in appearance of the hamartomatous components of the lesion with the various areas of the normal tracheobronchial tree. According to which, Type I, II, and III CCAM composed of bronchial/bronchiolar, bronchiolar, and bronchiolar/alveolar duct like structures, respectively. In 2002, Stocker himself revised this classification to include a total of five types by the addition of two more types, and changed the name of the disease from CCAM to CPAM [6]. The additional types were Type 0, which composed of tracheobronchial-like structures, and Type 4, which composed of thin-walled structures lined by alveolar lining cells, suggesting a malformation of the distal acinar components. Stocker specified the change from Roman to Arabic numerals for the revised classification in order to name the lesions of the proximal airway as "Type 0," that develop at an earlier stage than Type I, as the Roman numerals do not include zero [6].

In terms of the histological characteristics, CPAM Type 0 lesions exhibit irregular cartilage growth and immature mesenchymal tissue; Type 1 lesions contain mucus-producing cells; in Type 2 lesions, the cyst walls contain striated muscle; Type 3 lesions have the appearance of adenomatoid lobar tissue; and Type 4 lesions have the alveolar tissue stretched to varying degrees [6].

## 8.4 Prevalence

The reported incidence is between 1 in 10,000 and 1 in 35,000 with no predilection for side of lung, sex, or race [7, 8]. Since airway obstruction in fetal period is one of the leading etiologies for cystic lesions, the pathophysiology of congenital cystic lung disease (CCLD) has been recently reconsidered. Therefore, congenital cystic lesions that were formerly regarded as primary lesions may include many secondary cystic lesions associated with airway obstruction during the fetal lung development [9, 10]. As this new concept of the disease becomes more widespread, it is likely to affect the epidemiological frequency of CPAM, including the incidence of the different types. In terms of the incidence of the various types of CPAM, with respect to the new concept of the disease, Type 1 is understood to be the most common. Many of the lesions formerly classified as Type 2 were in fact secondary cystic lesions associated with bronchial atresia (BA) [9], while the actual Type 2 lesions only account for less than 30% of the cases. Additionally, Type 3, which was already known to be uncommon, accounts for approximately 10%, while Type 0 and Type 4 are extremely rare, accounting for less than 1% of

**Table 8.1** Characteristic of the patients with CPAM (1995–2018, at Osaka University Hospital and Osaka Women's and Children's Hospital)

| | Number of patients (%) ($n = 60$) |
|---|---|
| Gender (Male) | 35 (58%) |
| Prenatal diagnosis | 46 (77%) |
| Type (CPAM 1/CPAM 2/ CPAM 3) | 38 (63%)/17 (28%)/5 (8%) |
| Laterality (Right) | 33 (55%) |
| Lobe distribution (Upper/ Middle/Lower) | 15 (25%)/7 (12%)/38 (63%) |
| Surgery in neonatal period | 26 (43%) |
| Surgical procedure (Segmentectomy/Lobectomy) | 8 (13%)/52 (87%) |
| Surgical approach (Thoracoscopic/Open thoracotomy) | 5 (8%)/55 (92%) |
| Outcome (Survive) | 59 (98%) |

the cases [11]. Infants with CPAM accounted for 60 (32%) of the 188 infants with CCLD treated at Osaka University Hospital and Osaka Women's and Children's Hospital between 1995 and 2018. Among these 60 infants, 38 were diagnosed with CPAM Type 1 (63%), 17 with Type 2 (28%), and 5 with Type 3 (8%) (Table 8.1).

## 8.5 Differences Between CPAM and Other CCLDs

Because the diseases grouped under CCLD have different etiologies, CPAM differs both anatomically and pathophysiologically from other forms of CCLD such as BA and bronchopulmonary sequestration (BPS), which are also treated surgically. When considering the indications, timing, procedure, and other aspects of surgery for CPAM, it is imperative to appropriately understand the anatomical and pathophysiological differences between CPAM and other CCLDs.

### 8.5.1 Anatomical Differences

The primary anatomical difference is that there are no communications between the cystic lesions and the normal airways in BA, intralobular BPS, or extralobular BPS; however, the cystic lesions are communicated with the normal airways in CPAM. In BA and intralobular BPS, the affected lesions that are separated from the normal airways contain emphysematous lung tissues, caused by the trapped air that has entered from collateral ventilation and could not be expired through the normal airways. Although the isolated emphysematous lung tissue seen in BA or intralobular BPS do not expand beyond a certain size, there is a risk of unlimited distention of the cystic lesions in CPAM that are communicated with the normal airways, when filled with air upon spontaneous respiration or forced ventilation.

### 8.5.2 Pathophysiological Differences

In fetal lung development, alveolar fluid is produced by the alveolar epithelium. Because the affected lesion in BA and BPS are not communicated with the normal airways, they expand due to the retention of alveolar fluid between the 20th and 25th gestational week, compressing the normal lung. However, after the 28th gestational week the thoracic cavity and normal lung develop faster and grow larger than the expanded affected lesion, and thus the lesions become relatively smaller and this relieves the compression of the normal lung [1, 2, 12].

The amniotic fluid is moved in and out of the fetal airways and lungs as a result of fetal breathing movements in utero. It is speculated that the lesions of CPAM, that have expanded by the same process as in BA, are also filled with amniotic fluid by these fetal breathing movements, ensuing their expansion further given the communications between these lesions and the normal airways. Thus, lesions seen in the prenatal CPAM patients are generally larger compared with those in BA and BPS patients [13], and there is a lesser chance for them to shrink toward the end of gestation [3, 13, 14]. Therefore, neonates with CPAM tend to be associated with pulmonary hypoplasia of the normal lungs and often develop persistent pulmonary hypertension of the newborn (PPHN), that result in a high risk of

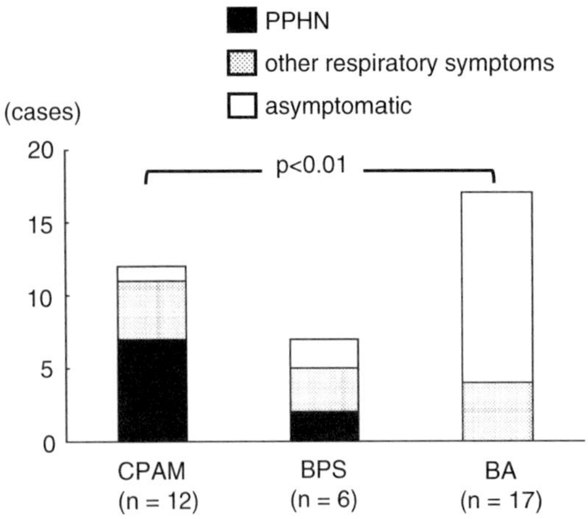


**Fig. 8.1** Respiratory symptoms of the neonates with congenital cystic lung diseases who were prenatally diagnosed at Osaka University Hospital between 1993 and 2013. *PPHN* persistent pulmonary hypertension of the newborn, *CPAM* congenital pulmonary airway malformation, *BPS* bronchopulmonary sequestration, *BA* bronchial atresia

severe postnatal respiratory impairment [15] (Fig. 8.1).

According to postnatal pathophysiology, CPAM lesions are more likely to be infected than those of BA or intralobular BPS. This is also because of the communications between the cystic lesions and the normal airways, that allows external pathogens to enter and lodge within the lesions.

## 8.6 Symptoms and Pathophysiology

In severe cases with a prenatal diagnosis, serious respiratory failure with cyanosis and bradycardia can occur immediately after birth, as may tachypnea, retractive breathing, and other symptoms of respiratory distress. Such severe cases of CPAM are believed to have pulmonary hypoplasia due to the mass effect of the lesions in utero. In CPAM Type 1 patients with huge cysts, a procedure known as thoracoamniotic shunting is performed in utero to prevent pulmonary hypoplasia [16].

Infants with severe CPAM often develop PPHN in the neonatal period. Once PPHN develops, the pulmonary artery goes into spasm, increasing pulmonary vascular resistance and causing right-to-left shunt via the ductus arteriosus. Thus, the systemic venous blood does not pass through the lungs and is not oxygenated before being recirculated, causing hypoxemia and acidosis. While the right-to-left shunt persists in the ductus arteriosus, the right ventricular afterload is reduced even if PPHN has developed. However, once the ductus arteriosus closes there is nowhere for the pressure from the right ventricle to be released and the right ventricular afterload increases, increasing the risk of a right cardiac failure.

Although congenital diaphragmatic hernia is a similar disorder which is also associated with pulmonary hypoplasia and PPHN, there is a difference between their clinical courses. In congenital diaphragmatic hernia, the PPHN improves over time and the patient's respiratory condition stabilizes, whereas in CPAM the patient's respiratory condition progressively worsen as the cystic lesions continue to expand upon taking in more air.

However, in mild cases with small lesions, even those diagnosed prenatally, no respiratory symptoms may occur postnatally, and the patient may remain asymptomatic. These asymptomatic cases are revealed when the cystic lesions become infected. A study found that 86% of prenatally diagnosed asymptomatic cases subsequently develop respiratory symptoms [17]. Japanese multicenter collaborative research reported that 68% of the prenatally diagnosed infants with CCLD including CPAM were asymptomatic after birth, but 85% of the asymptomatic cases develop respiratory symptoms thereafter [18].

## 8.7 Neonatal Onset Cases

### 8.7.1 Perioperative Management for Neonatal Onset Cases

The mainstay of circulatory management in severe cases of neonatal onset is the treatment for PPHN and right cardiac failure. PPHN should be treated by inhalation of nitric oxide (iNO) which selectively reduces pulmonary vascular resistance and increases pulmonary circulation volume. The iNO causes both increased oxygenation of blood and reduced afterload on the right ventricle. While pulmonary vascular resistance exceeds systemic vascular resistance, prostaglandin E1 is preferably administered to maintain the patency of ductus arteriosus, in order to reduce right ventricular afterload and maintain the systemic circulation by the cardiac output from the left ventricle. In rare cases, the use of extracorporeal membrane oxygenation may be required in patients associated with severe PPHN.

### 8.7.2 Surgical Treatment for Neonatal Onset Cases

Surgical treatment during the neonatal period is necessary for the infants with CPAM who reveal any respiratory symptoms after birth. Emergent resection of the cystic lung is required especially in cases showing severe respiratory distress immediately after birth. Additionally, patients in whom the cyst size increases rapidly due to mechanical ventilation or those in whom tension pneumothorax occurred by a rupture of the cyst may require an emergent thoracic drainage prior to the surgery [19] (Fig. 8.2).

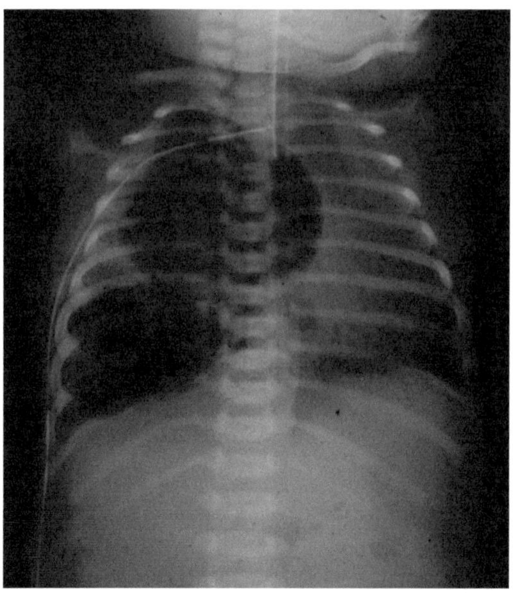

**Fig. 8.2** A 0-day-old boy of congenital pulmonary airway malformation Type 1. A chest tube was inserted into the right thoracic cavity prior to the surgery

However, during the operation, the cysts may rapidly increase in size by the inflow of air from the normal airway to the cysts, when positive pressure ventilation is initiated for general anesthesia. In such cases, pulmonary resection should be performed without delay with the assistance of inserting a tube into the cyst or a fenestration of the cyst to prevent the lesion from becoming enlarged during surgery.

## 8.8 Asymptomatic or Postnatal Onset Cases

### 8.8.1 Surgical Indications for Asymptomatic Cases

Surgery should be considered even in the asymptomatic cases of CPAM at birth in order to prevent respiratory infection, as it is reported that the lesions become infected in 23–89% of the patients [17, 20–22]. Given the possibility of the malignant tumor growth in the cystic lesion, surgery is also indicated for asymptomatic patients with CPAM [20, 23]. Removing the nonfunctional affected lesion in CPAM during infancy is also believed to be effective in creating space within the thoracic cavity for the expected growth of the normal lung.

### 8.8.2 Timing of Surgery for Asymptomatic Cases

Although patients with asymptomatic CPAM can be scheduled for an elective surgery, an optimal timing of surgery is still controversial. Since, in case of an infected cystic lesion, the inflammation tends to spread to the surrounding normal lung tissue, some insist that patients with CPAM who have been diagnosed prenatally, should undergo surgery within 3–6 months of their birth, prior to the onset of an infection [17, 22]. It is reported that elective resection including both open and thoracoscopic resection for the infants with asymptomatic CPAM are equally safe in 1–12 months of age [24, 25]. On the contrary, some others have a different opinion to wait until later childhood based on the long-term outcome. Follow-up findings showed better height and weight growth in patients operated upon in later childhood compared with those operated upon in infancy [26].

### 8.8.3 Surgery for Postnatal Onset Cases

Although some asymptomatic cases are diagnosed accidentally, such as when a patient undergoes an X-ray for a different reason, most postnatal onset cases are first identified when a lesion becomes infected. In the patients in whom the lesion is discovered due to an infection, the infection should be first controlled by conservative therapy and pulmonary resection should be performed after both the infection has resolved and the inflammation has subsided. Since the infection can recrudesce during the waiting period for a recovery from inflammation, it is important to perform the surgery opportunistically without delay. Patients who develop an infection may have severe adhesions and are likely to bleed; therefore, caution is required during the pulmonary resections.

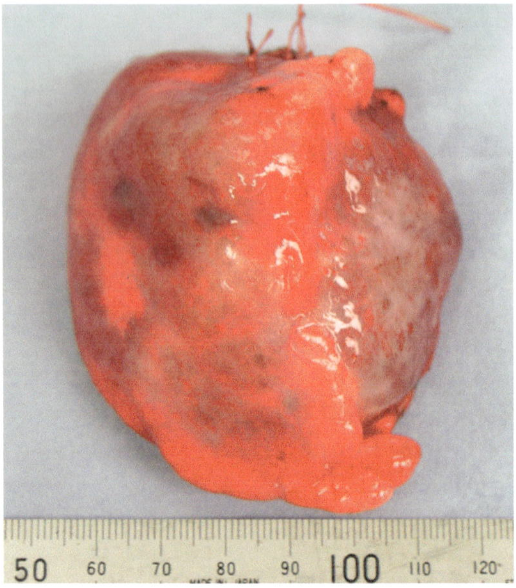

**Fig. 8.3** A specimen of lobectomy from a 0-day-old boy of congenital pulmonary airway malformation Type 2

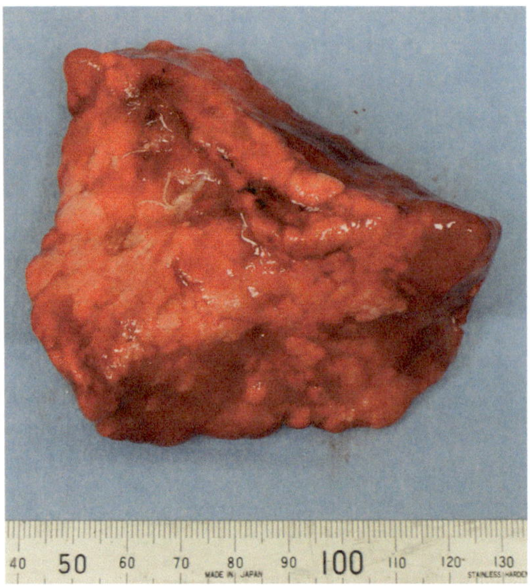

**Fig. 8.4** A specimen of lobectomy from a 1-day-old boy of congenital pulmonary airway malformation Type 3

## 8.9 Selection of Surgical Procedures

The selection of the procedure for pulmonary resection is important in CPAM patients. If the cystic lesion is located within a single lobe of the lung, lobectomy is usually preferred (Figs. 8.3 and 8.4). If the lesion is confined to several lung segments, segmentectomy can be performed [27, 28]. But in many cases CPAM lesions extend across the border of the segment, and the strategy must be to choose a surgical procedure that does not leave any residual lesions [29, 30].

The affected lesions may be present in multiple lobes in some CPAM cases. In such cases, given the priority to not have any residual lesions, unilateral total pneumonectomy might be the only choice. However, when total pneumonectomy is performed in infants it can result in complications with serious respiratory distress such as right pneumonectomy syndrome [31]. Therefore, performing total pneumonectomy in a single procedure should be avoided as much as possible, and the resection must be performed in stages, sparing at least one lobe even if this leaves some residual lesions.

## 8.10 Surgical Approach and Technique

Pulmonary resection in infants and children was previously performed via open surgery; however, in recent times, thoracoscopic surgery is being widely accepted for pulmonary resection in this patients population [32–34]. Thoracoscopic surgery requires technical and cognitive experience. Besides thorough knowledge of anatomy and anesthesia skills, the operator requires skills in minimally invasive surgery. Thus, a patient's age and the surgeon's expertise determine the choice between thoracotomy and thoracoscopy.

The primary difference between pulmonary resection performed for CPAM and procedures performed for other CCLDs is that the cystic lesions may progressively expand during the operation because the cystic lesions communicate with the patient's normal airway, and air enters the cysts during induction of general anesthesia secondary to positive pressure ventilation. Cyst expansion can interfere with the operative field; however, this technical obstacle can be overcome by ventilation of only the contralateral lung using differential lung ventilation or using a balloon to block the main bronchus of the ipsilateral lung being resected. However, if air continues to enter the cystic lesion causing them to enlarge, drain insertion into the cyst or cyst fenestration may enable effective continuous intraoperative decompression. Collapsing large cysts by the use of vessel-sealing device may also be effective to secure the operative field.

Unlike malignant tumor resection, tumor cell dissemination is not a concern in these cases. It should be remembered that when transecting blood vessels, the pulmonary arteries should be ligated and divided before the pulmonary veins to prevent vascular congestion of the lung. If all cystic parts of the CPAM are not treated, the residual cysts could act as a nidus for postoperative infection. Therefore, all affected lesions must be completely resected without any residual lesions [29, 30]. CPAM is often associated with incomplete interlobular fissures; therefore, interlobular dissection may be required, and the surgeon must ensure complete resection without any residual lesions.

## 8.11 Outcome

Excluding critically ill infants who require surgery immediately after birth, most infants with CPAM show a high survival rate. Although Type 3 CPAM was previously considered to be associated with poor prognosis [35], the mortality rate associated with this condition is lower than expected. Among 60 infants CPAM treated at Osaka University Hospital and Osaka Women's and Children's Hospital between 1995 and 2018, 26 (43%) infants underwent surgery during the neonatal period because of some respiratory symptoms after birth. Only 1 of the 60 (1.7%) infants died, who had Type 1 CPAM and underwent surgery during the neonatal period (Table 8.1). Watanabe et al. reported that among 37 infants with prenatally diagnosed CPAM, 10 (27%) patients were associated with fetal hydrops, 28 (76%) patients underwent emergent neonatal surgery and 32 (86%) patients survived [15]. Japanese multicenter collaborative research reported that among 243 neonates with CCLD including CPAM, 78 (32%) patients were symptomatic in neonatal period and 8 (3%) patients died [18]. It is also reported that the overall survival rate for 428 patients with CCLD including CPAM was 97% [18]. Nearly all infants who were asymptomatic during the neonatal period survived. Infants who survive postoperatively show favorable long-term prognosis [36].

## 8.12 Complications

Infants with large-volume lesions in utero often develop fetal hydrops (Fig. 8.5) and pulmonary hypoplasia before birth and are predisposed to PPHN after birth with long-term respiratory impairment postoperatively. Early postoperative

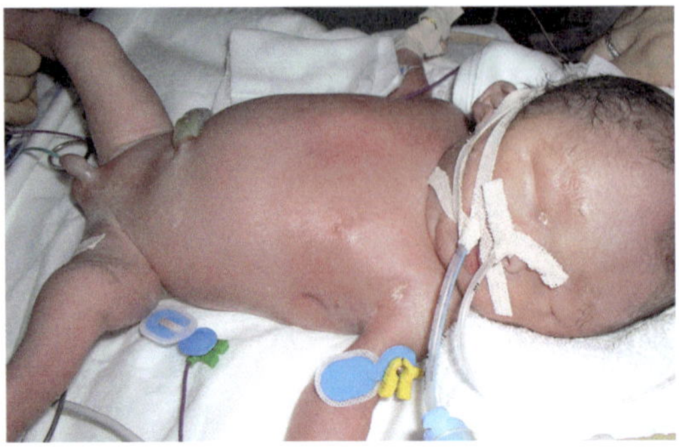

**Fig. 8.5** A 0-day-old boy of congenital pulmonary airway malformation Type 2 presented with a fetal hydrops

complications of CPAM include pneumothorax, atelectasis, pleural effusion, pneumonia, empyema, and persisting cystic lesion [18]. Late postoperative complications include thoracic deformity, persisting cystic lesion, chronic respiratory impairment, and growth retardations [18]. Infants with postoperative persisting cystic lesions may show recurrent CPAM with cyst enlargement.

Reportedly, several infants with CPAM often develop pectus excavatum before surgery [37], similar to the presentation of other CCLDs. Several infants also develop pectus excavatum postoperatively [37], and those who undergo open surgery during neonatal period or early infancy are particularly at a high risk of developing thoracic deformity as they grow. Pectus excavatum can be attributed to the fact that infants with CPAM develop retractive breathing continuously during infancy and early childhood, which exerts negative pressure on the anterior chest wall during inspiration.

Although malignant tumor such as pleuropulmonary blastoma may originate from the cystic lesions in infants with CPAM, whether CPAM predisposes to malignancy remains controversial, because it is likely that pleuropulmonary blastoma with cyst formation may initially have been misdiagnosed as CPAM [38]. However, there are several reports that CPAM were associated with malignant tumor such as pleuropulmonary blastoma and mucinous adenocarcinoma [20, 39].

## References


1. Illanes S, Hunter A, Evans M, et al. Prenatal diagnosis of echogenic lung: evolution and outcome. Ultrasound Obstet Gynecol. 2005;26:145–9.
2. Kunisaki SM, Barnewolt CE, Estroff JA, et al. Large fetal congenital cystic adenomatoid malformations: growth trends and patient survival. J Pediatr Surg. 2007;42:404–10.
3. Hadchouel A, Benachi A, Revillon Y, et al. Factors associated with partial and complete regression of fetal lung lesions. Ultrasound Obstet Gynecol. 2011;38:88–93.
4. Leblanc C, Baron M, Desselas E, et al. Congenital pulmonary airway malformations: state-of-the-art review for pediatrician's use. Eur J Pediatr. 2017;176:1559–71.
5. Stocker JT, Madewell JE, Drake RM. Congenital cystic adenomatoid malformation of the lung. Classification and morphologic spectrum. Hum Pathol. 1977;8:155–71.
6. Stocker JT. Congenital pulmonary airway malformation – a new name for and an expanded classification of congenital cystic adenomatoid malformation of the lung. Histopathology. 2002;41(Suppl. 2):424–31.
7. Prima FAFD, Bellia A, Inclimona G, et al. Antenatally diagnosed congenital cystic adenomatoid malformations (CCAM): research review. J Prenat Med. 2012;6:22–30.
8. Durell J, Lakhoo K. Congenital cystic lesions of the lung. Early Hum Dev. 2014;90:935–9.
9. Riedlinger WFJ, Vargas SO, Jennings RW, et al. Bronchial atresia is common to extralobar sequestration, intralobar sequestration, congenital cystic adenomatoid malformation, and lobar emphysema. Pediatr Develop Pathol. 2006;9:361–73.
10. Kunisaki SM, Fauza DO, Nemes LP, et al. Bronchial atresia: the hidden pathology within a spectrum of prenatally diagnosed lung masses. J Pediatr Surg. 2006;41:61–5.
11. Laje P, Liechty KW. Postnatal management and outcome of prenatally diagnosed lung lesions. Prenat Diagn. 2008;28:612–8.
12. Kunisaki SM, Buchner SE, Dillman JR, et al. Vanishing fetal lung malformations: prenatal sonographic characteristics and postnatal outcomes. J Pediatr Surg. 2015;50:978–82.
13. Kuroda T, Nishijima E, Maeda K, et al. Perinatal features of congenital cystic lung diseases: results of a nationwide multicentric study in Japan. Pediatr Surg Int. 2016;32:827–31.
14. Kuroda T, Morikawa N, Kitano Y, et al. Clinicopathologic assessment of prenatally diagnosed lung diseases. J Pediatr Surg. 2006;41:2028–31.
15. Watanabe T, Ohno M, Tahara K, et al. An investigation on clinical differences between congenital pulmonary airway malformation and bronchial atresia. J Pediatr Surg. 2018;53:2390–3.

16. Nitta H, Taira Y, Kinjo T, et al. Fetal thoracoamniotic shunting in a case of congenital pulmonary airway malformations with hydrops fetalis. Am J Perinatol Rep. 2017;7:e185–7.
17. Wong A, Vieten D, Singh S, et al. Long-term outcome of asymptomatic patients with congenital cystic adenomatoid malformation. Pediatr Surg Int. 2009;25:479–85.
18. Kuroda T, Nishijima E, Maeda K, et al. Clinical features of congenital cystic lung diseases: a report on a nationwide multicenter study in Japan. Eur J Pediatr Surg. 2016;26:91–5.
19. Oh SH, Kim CY, Lee BS, et al. Transthoracic catheter drainage for large symptomatic congenital pulmonary airway malformation. Pediatr Pulmolog. 2017;52:1572–7.
20. Durell J, Thakkar H, Gould S, et al. Pathology of asymptomatic, prenatally diagnosed cystic lung malformations. J Pediatr Surg. 2016;51:231–5.
21. Criss CN, Musili N, Matusko N, et al. Asymptomatic congenital lung malformations: is nonoperative management a viable alternative? J Pediatr Surg. 2018;53:1092–7.
22. Calvert JK, Lakhoo K. Antenatally suspected congenital cystic adenomatoid malformation of the lung: postnatal investigation and timing of surgery. J Pediatr Surg. 2007;2:411–4.
23. Morini F, Zani A, Conforti A, et al. Current management of congenital pulmonary airway malformations: a "European Pediatric Surgeons' Association" survey. Eur J Pediatr Surg. 2018;28:1–5.
24. Jelin EB, O'Hare EM, Jancelewic T, et al. Optimal timing for elective resection of asymptomatic congenital pulmonary airway malformations. J Pediatr Surg. 2018;53:1001–5.
25. Style CC, Cass DL, Verla MA, et al. Early vs late resection of asymptomatic congenital lung malformations. J Pediatr Surg. 2019;54:70–4.
26. Pinter A, Kalman A, Karsza L, et al. Long-term outcome of congenital cystic adenomatoid malformation. Pediatr Surg Int. 1999;15:332–5.
27. Bagrodia N, Cassel S, Liao J, et al. Segmental resection for the treatment of congenital pulmonary malformations. J Pediatr Surg. 2014;49:905–9.
28. Kim HK, Choi YS, Kim K, et al. Treatment of congenital cystic adenomatoid malformation: should lobectomy always be performed? Ann Thorac Surg. 2008;86:249–53.
29. Khosa JK, Leong SL, Borzi PA. Congenital cystic adenomatoid malformation of the lung: indications and timing of surgery. Pediatr Surg Int. 2004;20:505–8.
30. Luja'n M, Bosque M, Mirapeix RM, et al. Late-onset congenital cystic adenomatoid malformation of the lung. Respiration. 2002;69:148–54.
31. Stolar BC, Berdon W, Reyes C. Right pneumonectomy syndrome: a lethal complication of lung resection in a newborn with cystic adenomatoid malformation. J Pediatr Surg. 1988;12:1180–3.
32. Nasr A, Bass J. Thoracoscopic vs open resection of congenital lung lesions: a meta-analysis. J Pediat Surg. 2012;47:857–61.
33. Polites SF, Habermann EB, Zarroug AZ. Thoracoscopic vs open resection of congenital cystic lung diseaseutilization and outcomes in 1120 children in the United States. J Pediatr Surg. 2016;51:1101–5.
34. Adams S, Jobson M, Sangnawakij P. Does thoracoscopy have advantages over open surgery for asymptomatic congenital lung malformations? An analysis of 1626 resections. J Pediatr Surg. 2017;52:247–51.
35. Sakala EP, Perrott WS, Grube GL. Sonographic characteristics of antenatally diagnosed extralobar pulmonary sequestration and congenital cystic adenomatoid malformation. Obstet Gynecol Surv. 1994;49:647–55.
36. Tsai AY, Liechty KW, Hedrick HL. Outcomes after postnatal resection of prenatally diagnosed asymptomatic cystic lung lesions. J Pediatr Surg. 2008;43:513–7.
37. Delestrain C, Khen-Dunlop N, Hadchouel A, et al. Respiratory morbidity in infants born with a congenital lung malformation. Pediatrics. 2017;139:e20162988. https://doi.org/10.1542/peds.2016-2988.
38. Feinberg A, Hall NJ, Williams GM, et al. Can congenital pulmonary airway malformation be distinguished from type I pleuropulmonary blastoma based on clinical and radiological features? J Pediar Surg. 2016;51:33–17.
39. Koh J, Jung E, Jan SJ, et al. A case of mucinous adenocarcinoma of the lung associated with congenital pulmonary airway malformation in a neonate. Korean J Pediatr. 2018;61:30–4.

# 9 Surgical Treatment for Bronchial Obstruction

Hiroomi Okuyama

**Abstract**

Bronchial atresia (BA) is a rare congenital pulmonary disorder characterized by mucinous cyst and peripheral emphysematous lesion. The numbers of prenatally diagnosed BA have increased in recent years. The typical CT findings include occlusions of the bronchus central to the mucocele, emphysematous changes of the peripheral lung fields. CPAM lesion is often associated with the peripheral area of the atretic bronchus. Clinical presentation is widely variable, ranging from asymptomatic to life-threatening. Although the most common surgical indication is recurrent infection, surgery on asymptomatic cases remains controversial. The long-term outcome is excellent if the residual lung function is well preserved after operation.

**Keywords**

Congenital bronchial atresia · Congenital cystic lung disease · CAPM · Prenatal diagnosis · Emphysema · Bronchocele Surgery

Congenital bronchial atresia (BA), first reported by Ramsay in 1953 [1], is a rare congenital pulmonary disorder characterized by mucinous cyst and peripheral emphysematous; this is partly due to the proximal segmental or lobar bronchus involved obstruction, resulted in a mucus-filled bronchocele in a distal end of segmental or lobar bronchus and local emphysema formed by collateral ventilation air (Fig. 9.1).

The precise pathogenesis of this disease is unclear. The process of the normal airway development is completed by the 16 weeks of gestational age. As the bronchial pattern distal to the site of atresia is normal, it is speculated that the atresia is not a result of normal growth failure but is secondary to a traumatic insult of fetal life after 16th week. One theory is there has been occlusion of the blood supply to the affected bronchus after the normal airway development [2].

While BA is congenital, the onset time differs depending on each case. A review of the reported cases indicates that over half present in patients under 15 years of age [3]. Although there is no consensus on the site of lesion, it has been reported that CBA frequently affects the left upper lobe [4]. However, another research found that the right lung is the most common site [5].

H. Okuyama (✉)
Department of Pediatric Surgery, Osaka University Graduate School of Medicine, Osaka, Japan
e-mail: okuyama@pedsurg.med.osaka-u.ac.jp





H. Sago et al. (eds.), *Congenital Cystic Lung Disease*, https://doi.org/10.1007/978-981-15-5175-8_9

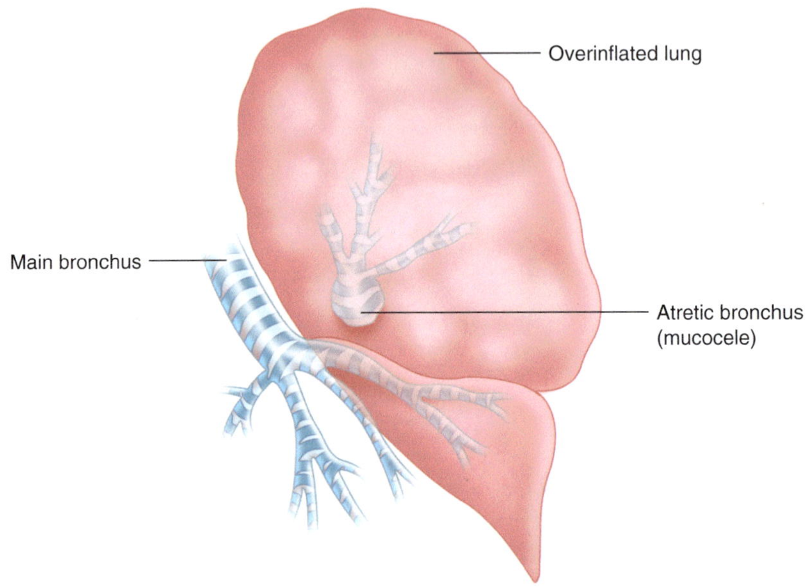


**Fig. 9.1** A typical form of bronchial atresia associated with mucocele and overinflated lung

## 9.1 Classifications

There are two types of BA based on the site of the atresia; proximal/peripheral:

1. Proximal atresia is located at the level of the mainstem or the proximal lobar bronchi, which is extremely rare and usually lethal during pregnancy. Proximal atresia causes a tremendous volume increase of the distal involved lung with secondary hypoplasia of the normal lung. According to a review of seven cases of main bronchial atresia, five cases were stillbirth or immediate death after birth and the remaining two cases were dead after pneumonectomy [6].
2. Peripheral atresia is located at the segmental/subsegmental bronchial level, which may present as an isolated lesion or as part of a complex congenital malformation. Prenatal findings are mostly nonspecific. Therefore, bronchial atresia is rarely recognized prenatally. There are few case reports of prenatally diagnosed peripheral BA [7–9]. Postnatal exams show overinflated lung areas and focal bronchial dilations. The typical fluid-filled bronchoceles are not always observed in neonates but develop progressively in the first months of life. CPAM is often associated with the peripheral area of the atretic bronchus.

## 9.2 Clinical Presentation

**(Prenatal)**

The numbers of prenatal diagnosis and characterization of congenital lung malformations have increased in recent years due to the generalization and technical improvements of antenatal US and the use of MRI for select cases [10, 11]. Proximal atresia causes a huge volume increase of the distal involved lung, which appears homogeneously hyperechogenic at US. The mass effect of the abnormal lung usually causes eversion of the ipsilateral hemidiaphragm, mediastinal shift, and severe compression of the normal lung. A bronchocele, a centrally located, fluid-filled, tubular structure, is often observed and reflects the dilation of the bronchus distal to the atresia. Peripheral isolated atresia is difficult to identify in utero as most cases only show nonspecific imaging findings that reflect the impaired elimination of the pulmonary fluid distal to the obstruction level.

However, BA should be considered when CCAM type III was diagnosed prenatal by US. Bronchial dilations may also be present in peripheral bronchial atresia, but they are rarely detected prospectively because of their small size.

**(Postnatal)**

The postnatal course of those cases can also be widely variable, ranging from asymptomatic to life-threatening. Some cases of prenatally diagnosed BA are completely asymptomatic. In such cases, it is common to follow up for a while after birth. Surgery on those cases remains controversial. In contrast, some cases of prenatally diagnosed BA are life-threatening which require immediate intervention after birth. Seo et al. reported a neonatal BA case in which left upper pulmonary lobectomy was performed at 7 days of age because of respiratory distress caused by massive enlargement of the left upper lobe [8]. The most common clinical presentations of BA include recurrent pulmonary infection, wheezing, and respiratory distress. Patients who present with this condition beyond the first few weeks of life show hyperinflation or emphysema of the lung distal to the atresia. Air exchange through the pores of Kohn and the channels of Lambert explains air entry into the lung distal to the atresia. This collateral ventilation appears to be more effective on inspiration, and therefore, it maintains the inspiratory phase, giving it the roentgenographic appearance of hyperinflation with air trapping. A review of 29 BA patients aged from 1 day to 13 years revealed that the most frequent symptom was productive cough and fever owing to recurrent pneumonia found in 26 children [5]. There appears to be a progressive increase in symptoms secondary to episodes of infection in the lung involved in the atresia, as well as in adjacent pulmonary tissue compressed by the hyperinflated lung.

## 9.3 Diagnosis

A clinical diagnosis of BA mainly depends on a combination of CT and clinical pathologic diagnosis. Representative chest radiographs of BA show hyperinflated lung because the lung areas peripheral to the occlusion site exhibit overinflation or emphysema through the collateral ventilation. However, this finding is not specific to BA (Fig. 9.2).

CT is a very sensitive method for demonstrating the typical features of bronchial atresia. A plug of desquamated tissue and mucus filling the dilated bronchus distal to the point of atresia or stenosis appears to be an unvarying component of the syndrome and has been termed a "mucocele." The typical CT characteristics of bronchial atresia include occlusions of the bronchus central to the mucocele, emphysematous changes of the peripheral lung fields, and bronchogenic cyst (Fig. 9.3).

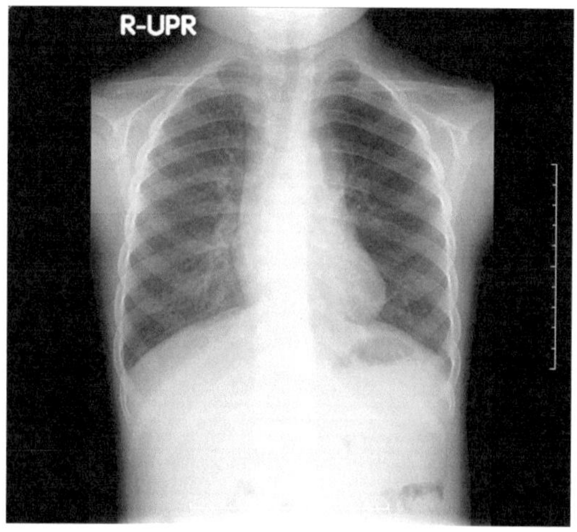


**Fig. 9.2** Left upper lesion is overinflated due to peripheral type of BA

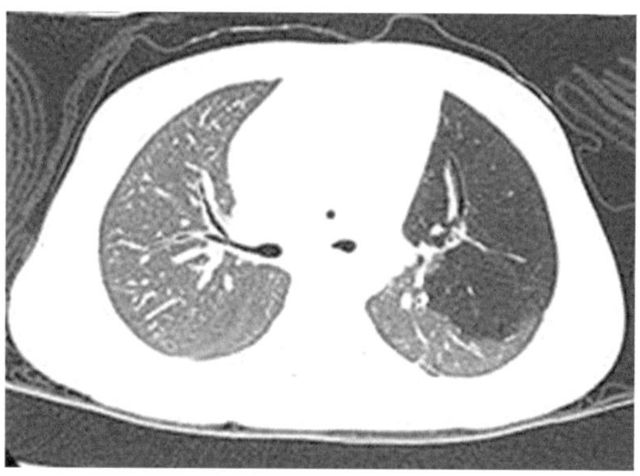

**Fig. 9.3** Emphysematous changes of the peripheral lung fields and dilated bronchus distal to the atretic bronchus) (same case as Fig. 9.2)

In some cases of BA, congenital pulmonary airway malformation (CPAM) lesion coexists. Figure 9.4 shows a cyst filled with mucous (mucocele) at the beginning of B6 and coexisting CPAM type2 lesion distal to the obstruction.

There are few reports of BA in which atelectasis and airless mass filled with fluid were observed (Fig. 9.5a, b).

Bronchofiberscopy (BF) is also helpful in identifying a blind-terminating bronchus. However, the role of BF for the diagnosis of peripheral BA in infants and children is limited. In many cases of peripheral BA in children, it is difficult to detect the atretic point directly by BF, because BF is thick and often cannot reach the atretic bronchus.

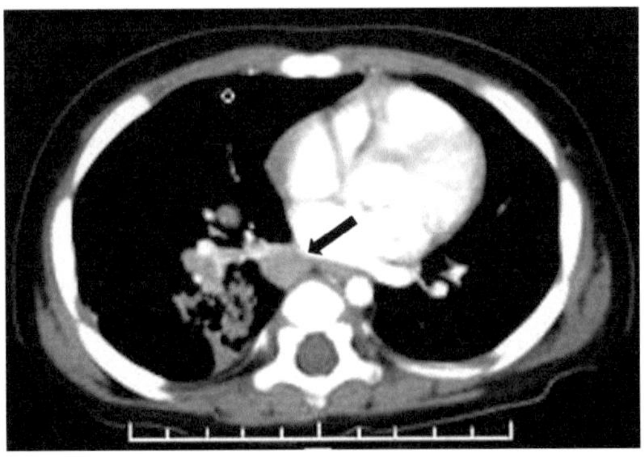

**Fig. 9.4** A cyst filled with mucous (mucocele) at the beginning of B6 (arrow) and coexisting CPAM type 2 lesion distal to the obstruction

Three-dimensional CT bronchography has recently been used for the evaluation of congenital tracheobronchial lesions and shows an absence of connection between the bronchus in the hyperinflated lobes or segments and the more proximal bronchus [8].

## 9.4 Treatment (Surgical and Medical)

There is significant debate regarding the treatment of BA. Some prefer to perform surgery on all patients. However, some publications advocated that surgery should be reserved only for patients with serious complications.

The surgical indications include: the patient has recurrent and severe infection symptoms (such as pneumonias, dyspnea, cough, or hemoptysis) and medical treatment ineffective; malignant lesions cannot be excluded.

As respiratory infection repeats, the extent of lung resection increases. Therefore, surgery before repeated infection is recommended to preserve the residual lung function as much as possible.

After thoracotomy, the affected side of the lung is blocked and collapsed. In patient with overinflated lesion, the affected segment can be easily recognized as the persistent emphysema (Fig. 9.6).

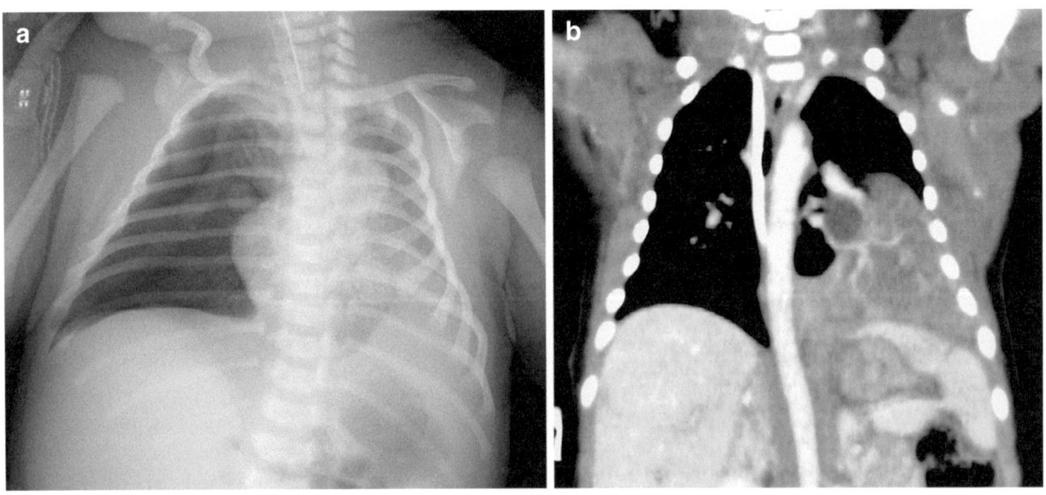


**Fig. 9.5** (**a**, **b**) A dilated bronchus filled with mucus (mucocele) and atelectasis distal to the atresia

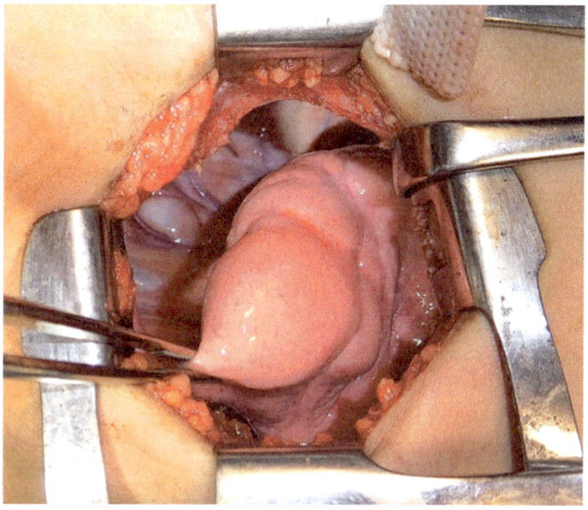

**Fig. 9.6** Persistent emphysema of the affected BA lesion (same case as Fig. 9.2)

To preserve the residual lung function, resection should be limited to the affected lesion as much as possible. In patients with peripheral BA, segmentectomy makes more sense than lobectomy.

In BA, the pulmonary vasculature is usually normal. Therefore, the first step of the operation is to identify and divide the pulmonary artery and vein of the BA segment as usual lung resection. In contrast, the operative findings of the atretic bronchus can be variable. In some cases, the atretic bronchus is occluded in the lumen with the normal continuity to the central bronchus. In other cases, the atretic bronchus is interrupted. Therefore, it is difficult to confirm the diagnosis of BA based on the operative findings.

Because such benign disease often occurs in young patients, minimally invasive surgery, such as thoracoscopic surgery, is recommended. Recent advancement of minimally invasive surgical techniques and instruments have made thoracoscopic lung resection a safe and feasible treatment even in small children. If possible, local resection should be performed as a first option, and on the basis of the intraoperative pathological results, a decision can be made regarding the need for further surgery. However, because lesions always invade the hilar region, it is very difficult to dissect the affected bronchial and pulmonary vessels, and local resection can be replaced by standard lobectomy.

## 9.5 Pathology

Diagnosis of BA can be confirmed by the pathological findings of a blind-ending bronchus associated with a distal mucous-filled bronchocele. The gross appearance of the surgical specimen usually reveals an overinflated lung with occasional subpleural blebs and sometimes grossly evident subpleural cystic areas. The bronchus lacks a proximal or central tracheal communication. Distal to the atresia there is cystic dilatation of the bronchus that contains plugs of desquamated tissue and mucus. The lining surfaces of the bronchi are smooth and thin-walled, and there may be absence of grossly evident cartilage. Microscopic examination shows dilatation of alveoli without destruction of alveolar walls. Many of the expanded alveoli have a cystic appearance.

## 9.6 Prognosis

Recently nonsurgical observation is increasing in asymptomatic cases in which prenatally diagnosis is made. To date, because long-term outcome of those asymptomatic cases is unclear, it is still controversial whether surgery is recommended for those asymptomatic cases or not.

In operation cases, the long-term outcome is excellent if the residual lung function is well preserved after operation. If multiple lesions exist, extensive lung resection aiming to complete removal of the lesions should be avoided.

## References


1. Ramsay BH. Mucocele of the lung due to congenital obstruction of a segmental bronchus; a case report; relationship to congenital cystic disease of the lung and to congenital bronchiectasis. Dis Chest. 1953;24:96–103.
2. Schuster SR, Harris GB, Williams A, Kirkpatrick J, Reid L. Bronchial atresia: a recognizable entity in the pediatric age group. J Pediatr Surg. 1978;13(6D):682–9.
3. Asada M, Yano S, Okayasu K, Tanabe T, Hiraga T, Kawakami Y. A case report of congenital bronchial

atresia – a review of 43 cases in Japan. Nihon Kyobu Geka Gakkai Zasshi. 1991;39(4):463.
4. Jederlinic PJ, Sicilian LS, Baigelman W, et al. Congenital bronchial atresia. A report of 4 cases and a review of the literature. Medicine (Baltimore). 1987;66:73–83.
5. Morikawa N, Kuroda T, Honna T, et al. Congenital bronchial atresia in infants and children. J Pediatr Surg. 2005;40:1822–6.
6. Zamora IJ, Sheikh F, Olutoye OO, et al. Mainstem bronchial atresia: a lethal anomaly amenable to fetal surgical treatment. J Pediatr Surg. 2014;49:706–11.
7. Kamata S, Sawai T, Usui N, Nose K, Kitayama Y, Iiboshi Y, Okada A, Kanzaki T. Case of congenital bronchial atresia detected by fetal ultrasound. Pediatr Pulmonol. 2003;35:227–9.
8. Seo T, Ando H, Kaneko K, Ono Y, Tainaka T, Sumida W, Hayakawa M, Itakura A. Two cases of prenatally diagnosed congenital lobar emphysema caused by lobar bronchial atresia. J Pediatr Surg. 2006;41:E17–20.
9. Alamo L, Vial Y, Carole Gengler C, Meuli R. Imaging findings of bronchial atresia in fetuses, neonates and infants. Pediatr Radiol. 2016;46:383–90.
10. Yu G, Xia B, Wang Z, Huang B, Zhang Y, Hong C, Shang N, Tang J. Prenatal and postnatal management of congenital bronchial atresia (CBA): single tertiary center report. J Matern Fetal Neonatal Med. 2017;30(16):2006–10.
11. Keswani SG, Crombleholme TM, Pawel BR, et al. Prenatal diagnosis and management of mainstem bronchial atresia. Fetal Diagn Ther. 2005;20:74–8.

# Intralobar Pulmonary Sequestration

10

Yutaka Kanamori

**Abstract**

Pulmonary sequestration is a congenital respiratory malformation characterized by a cystic or solid mass of nonfunctioning primitive segmental lung tissue that does not communicate with the tracheobronchial tree and has anomalous systemic blood supply. Pulmonary sequestration is classified into two types, extralobar pulmonary sequestration and intralobar pulmonary sequestration (ILS). ILS is incorporated within the normal lung tissue and does not have a visceral pleura that separates the lesion from normal lung tissue. Here the 35 pediatric ILS cases treated in our center are summarized first and then we review several clinical reports that dealt with ILS in the past and summarize the characters and treatment of ILS.

Patients with ILS show nonspecific respiratory symptoms such as cough, expectoration, hemoptysis, and chest pain. Recently the number of the cases with fetal diagnosis is increasing. The existence of an aberrant artery to the lung lesion from systemic circulation is an important finding for the correct diagnosis of ILS. The lobectomy including the affected lung is mandatory for complete cure and the prognosis of ILS is satisfactory after the proper surgical treatment.

**Keywords**

Intralobar pulmonary sequestration · Aberrant artery · Prenatal diagnosis · Fetal MRI · Fetal ultrasound examination · Lobectomy

## 10.1 Introduction

Pulmonary sequestration is a congenital respiratory malformation characterized by a cystic or solid mass of nonfunctioning primitive segmental lung tissue that does not communicate with the tracheobronchial tree and has anomalous systemic blood supply. Pulmonary sequestration was first reported more than 100 years ago. In 1946 Pryce [1] first used the term "sequestration" for this pathological state and classified it into two phenotypes of "intra" and "extra" pulmonary sequestration. Since then, pulmonary sequestration has come to be accepted as a distinct clinical entity.

Pulmonary sequestration is generally considered to be caused by a developmental anomaly occurring at an early gestational age and the sequestered lung tissue with a systemic arterial supply is formed independently of the normal lung. Pulmonary sequestration is not only anatomically distinct from normal lung tissue but

Y. Kanamori (✉)
Division of Surgery, Department of Surgical Specialties, National Center for Child Health and Development, Tokyo, Japan
e-mail: kanamori-y@ncchd.go.jp





H. Sago et al. (eds.), *Congenital Cystic Lung Disease*, https://doi.org/10.1007/978-981-15-5175-8_10

physiologically distinct, which means that the sequestered lung is not connected to the broncho-pulmonary system of the normal lung and has no gas exchange function.

Pulmonary sequestration is classified into two pathological entities: extralobar sequestration (ELS) and intralobar sequestration (ILS). Extralobar sequestration is defined as its boundary being separated from normal lung tissue by its own visceral pleura, and intralobar sequestration is incorporated within the normal lung tissue and does not have a visceral pleura that separates the lesion from normal lung tissue.

## 10.2 Our Cases

We present here the experience of our center in treating ILS surgically and discuss characteristics of the disease.

### 10.2.1 The Experience of Treatment of Pediatric ILS Cases in Our Center from 2002 to 2019

In 2015 we reported our experience of 30 pediatric ILS cases [2], and since then, we experienced another 5 cases. Here the 35 pediatric ILS cases treated in our center are summarized.

We experienced 35 pediatric cases of ILS from April 2002 to March 2019 that were treated by surgical removal of a pulmonary lobe including the sequestered lung tissue (Table 10.1).

There were 14 male patients and 21 female patients. The age at the time of the operation ranged from 5 months to 124 months (mean age, 32 months). All sequestered lungs were situated in the lower lung field; the sequestered lung was situated in the left lower lung in 17 cases and in the right lower lung in 18 cases. Fetal diagnosis was attained in 13 cases (37.1%), and its percentage has been increasing recently. Since 2014 we experienced five cases of ILS and all of them were diagnosed prenatally. The age at the time of the operation was younger in the cases with fetal diagnosis (mean age was 13 months, compared with a mean age of 42 months in the postnatally diagnosed cases). Twenty cases of ILS experienced pneumonia before the operation but no case showed respiratory distress in their daily life.

**Table 10.1** Patient characteristics ($n$ = 35)

| | |
|---|---|
| Gender | Male:Female = 14:21 |
| Affected side | Right:Left = 18:17 |
| Localization of the lesions | Lower lobe 35 (100%) |
| History of pulmonary infection | 20 (57%) |
| Prenatally diagnosed cases | 13 (37%) |
| Median age at the operation | 32 months |

The characteristics of the aberrant artery that supplied the sequestered lung in the 35 ILS cases are summarized. The aberrant artery branched from the thoracic aorta in 13 cases, from the abdominal aorta in 17 cases, and from the celiac artery in 5 cases (Fig. 10.1). Another important factor is the number of aberrant arteries. In our series, 31 cases had one aberrant artery, and 4 cases had two aberrant arteries (Fig. 10.1). Venous drainage from the sequestered lung is another important point (Table 10.2). In 32 cases, venous drainage was through the pulmonary vein on the affected side. In one case, venous drainage was through the inferior vena cava. The remaining two cases each had two drainage veins, i.e., through the pulmonary vein and the azygos vein.

The operative procedure was lower lobectomy by thoracotomy in all 35 cases. There were no complications experienced during and after the operation.

## 10.3 Previous Case Series

Pulmonary sequestration is a relatively rare disease, and a few case series [3–10] and review articles [11, 12] on pulmonary sequestration have been published that included adult cases only or both adult and pediatric cases. One review article that summarized Chinese cases of pulmonary sequestration [11] is the largest case review and it reported the characteristics of 2625 pulmonary sequestration cases. In their review, the male-to-female ratio was 1.58:1. The age of the patients at the time of the operation ranged from 1 month to 77 years, and the mean age at the time of the operation for ILS was younger than that for ELS (20 ± 8 years vs. 38 ± 9 years).

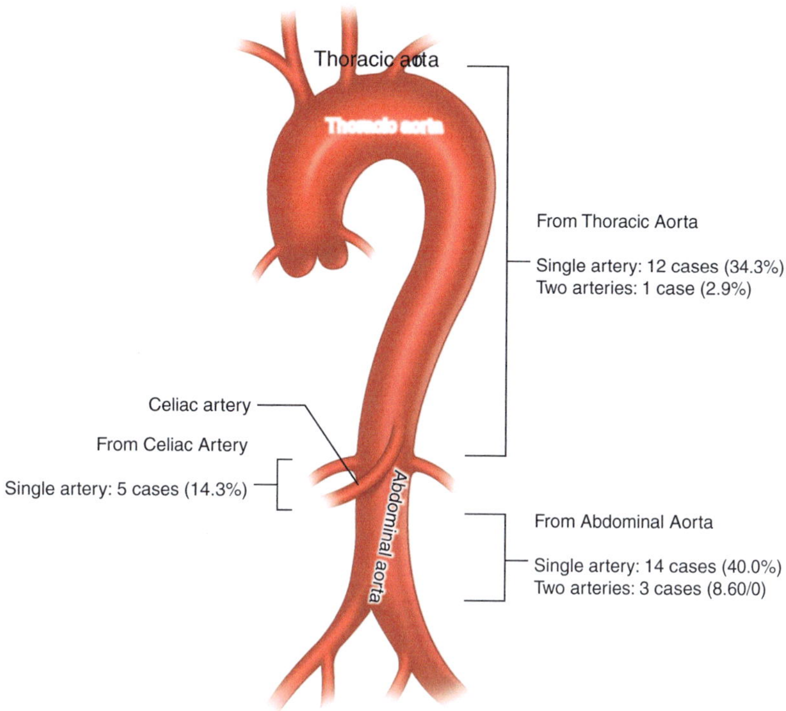


**Fig. 10.1** The route of the aberrant arteries to the sequestered lung in 35 cases of ILS treated at our hospital. A single aberrant artery was seen in 31 cases and two aberrant arteries were seen in 4 cases. The aberrant artery branched from the thoracic aorta in 13 cases, the abdominal aorta in 17 cases, and the celiac artery in 5 cases. Among the four cases with double aberrant arteries, one case had aberrant arteries branching from the thoracic aorta and three cases had aberrant arteries branching from the abdominal aorta

**Table 10.2** Drainage vein(s) from the sequestered lung segment

| | |
|---|---|
| To pulmonary vein only | 32 cases (91.4%) |
| To inferior vena cava | 1 case (2.9%) |
| To pulmonary vein and azygos vein | 2 cases (5.7%) |

The symptoms of the disease included cough/ expectoration (67.76%), fever (38.95%), hemoptysis (27.67%), and chest pain (11.13%).

## 10.4 Clinical Aspects

Image findings of chest computed tomography (CT) were classified as follows: mass lesion (49.01%), cystic lesion (28.57%) (Fig. 10.2a shows a typical image of a cystic lesion experienced in our center), cavity lesion (11.57%), pneumonic lesion (7.96%), and bronchiectasia (1.90%) (Fig. 10.2b shows a typical image of bronchiectasia experienced in our center). Among pulmonary sequestrations, unilateral ILS was the most common phenotype, accounting for 1873 cases (83.95%), and unilateral ELS accounted for 358 cases (16.05%). Bilateral lesions were extremely rare, with only three cases seen in the series from China. The sequestered lung was mainly localized in the left lower lobe (1457 cases; 71.53%), and the second common segment was the right lower lobe (529 cases; 25.97%). Other localized regions of sequestered lung were the left upper lobe, left lingual lobe, right upper lobe, and right middle lobe. In our experience, all lesions were situated in the lower lung segment, and the left-to-right ratio was about 1:1. ILS has a special feature compared with other congenital pulmonary cystic diseases such as congenital pulmonary airway malformation (CPAM) and bronchial atresia in that the lesion of ILS belongs to one area of the normal lung and single lobectomy is always possible for complete cure. Therefore, it is important to detect the exact site of the ILS lesion for proper surgical excision. ILS was also reported to coincide with other congenital anomalies [11] such as esophagobronchial diverticulum, diaphragmatic hernia [13], deformities of skeletal systems, and cardiac anom-

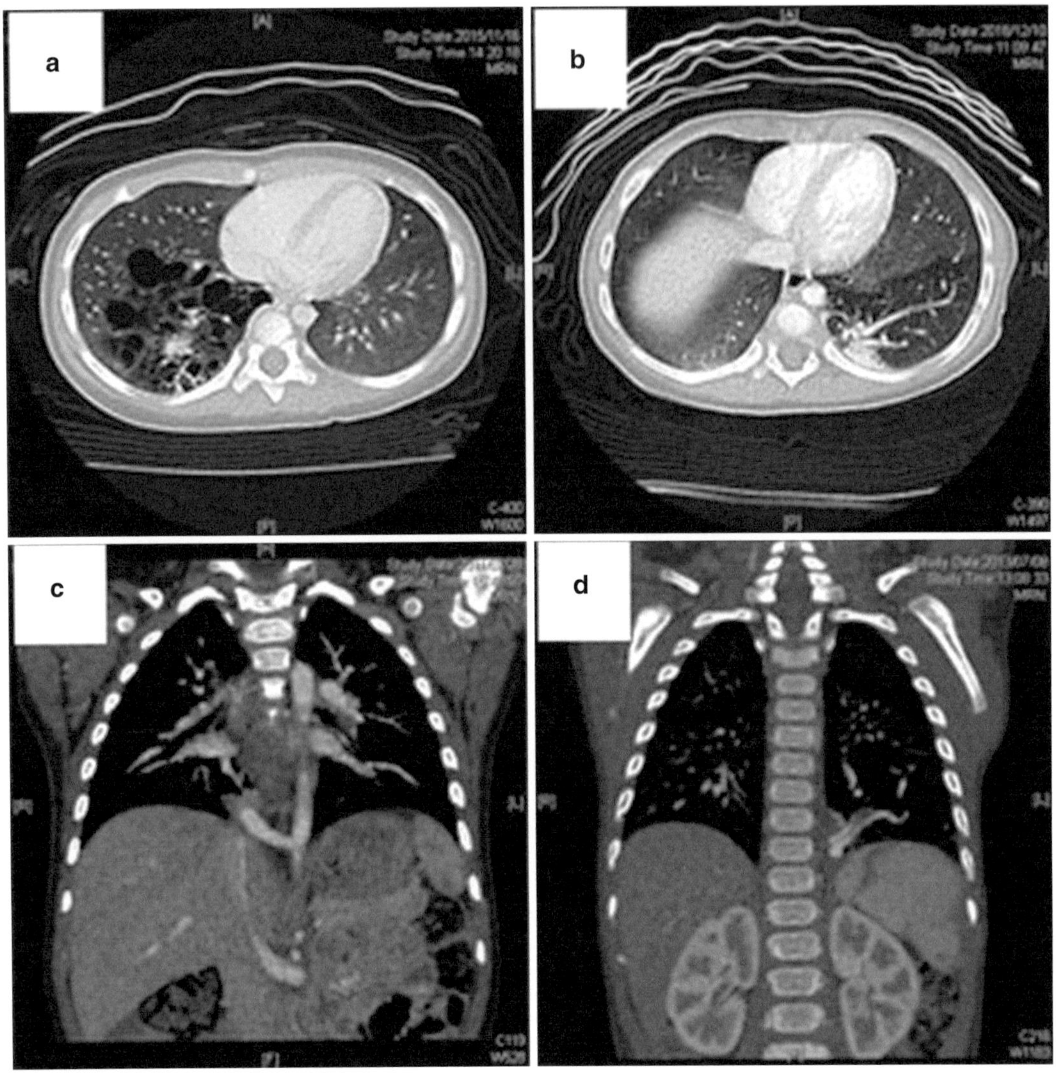


**Fig. 10.2** Representative CT findings of lung fields and aberrant arteries in ILS. (**a**) Cystic lesion, which represents the sequestered lung, in the right lower lobe. (**b**) Hyperlucent lesion, which represents the sequestered lung, in the left lower lobe. A large aberrant artery is seen running amidst the affected lung. (**c**) A large aberrant artery branched from the thoracic aorta to the sequestered lung in the right lower lobe. (**d**) Two aberrant arteries branched from the thoracic aorta to the sequestered lung in the left lower lobe

alies. Some case reports described the association of bronchogenic cyst with ILS [14].

The most important factor for safe treatment of ILS is determining the arterial supply and venous drainage of the sequestered lung. Detection of the aberrant artery is a key point for correct diagnosis of ILS [15–18], and preoperative confirmation of the blood supply and the drainage route is mandatory for carrying out a safe operative procedure.

On fetal ultrasound examination, if an abnormal pulmonary lesion is detected, it should be checked whether the systemic arterial supply to the lesion exists from the aorta or from one of its branches. Fetal magnetic resonance imaging (MRI) examination may be useful to confirm the abnormal arterial supply. If such abnormal arterial branch to the lesion is detected, pulmonary sequestration should be strongly suspected. On the other hand, it is also important to determine venous drainage from the lesion because in ILS venous drainage is mainly through the pulmonary vein while in ELS venous drainage is usually through a systemic route [11]. We must carefully differentiate ILS from ELS because in some ILS cases venous drainage is through a systemic vein such as the azygos vein, semi-azygos vein, or inferior vena cava. In our series, three cases had such systemic drainage. Postnatal chest CT examination may be able to demonstrate whether the pulmonary lesion has its own visceral pleura or not, and therefore may be useful to differentiate ILS from ELS.

It is important to recognize the symptoms of ILS, especially in adults, but disease-specific symptoms do not exist and almost all symptoms such as cough, expectoration, fever, hemoptysis, and chest pain are not specific [11]. Hemoptysis is in one sense a specific symptom of ILS but in pediatric cases it is rarely seen. In our series, pneumonia was a main symptom in obtaining a correct diagnosis before the fetal diagnostic era, but recently there has been a predominance of cases with fetal diagnosis and in many cases curative operation was performed before pneumonic symptoms appeared. Recent basic research suggested that in ILS alveolar type 2 stem/progenitor cells are impaired in their proliferative potential perhaps through the interaction between endothelial thrombospondin-1 and alveolar cell surface antigen CD36, and this may be closely related to the high infection rate in patients with ILS [19]. Blood tests in patients with ILS do not show specific abnormalities, but in some reports serum CA19-9 was elevated in patients with ILS and it significantly decreased after surgery [20, 21]. The exact mechanism of this phenomenon has not yet been clarified, but serum CA19-9 might be used as a disease marker of ILS in restricted cases. Especially in adults, when patients show a high level of CA19-9, ILS should be among the differential diagnoses after ruling out malignancies of digestive organs.

## 10.5 Treatment

The treatment strategy for ILS is surgical removal of the pulmonary lobe containing the sequestered lung once the diagnosis is confirmed. As ILS often causes respiratory infection and hemoptysis is a nuisance complication in later life, it is recommended that patients with ILS undergo the operative treatment. In some reports, embolization of the aberrant artery was successful and this is one treatment option [22–25]. Another interesting option for surgical resection of the small lesion is indocyanine green injection and navigated partial lung resection [26]. If the lesion is very small and it is desirable to preserve as much of the normal lung as possible, this strategy may be adopted. Recently video-assisted thoracoscopic surgery (VATS) and thoracoscopic surgery have become more popular and some reports recommended such minimally invasive surgery [7, 10]. In such procedure, safe dissection of a large aberrant artery is very important and skillful technique is mandatory for preventing severe bleeding complications. Another important point for performing safe surgery is accurate preoperative diagnosis concerning the aberrant artery (Figs. 10.2c, d and 10.3a–c) and the drainage vein (Fig. 10.4). In some cases, more than one

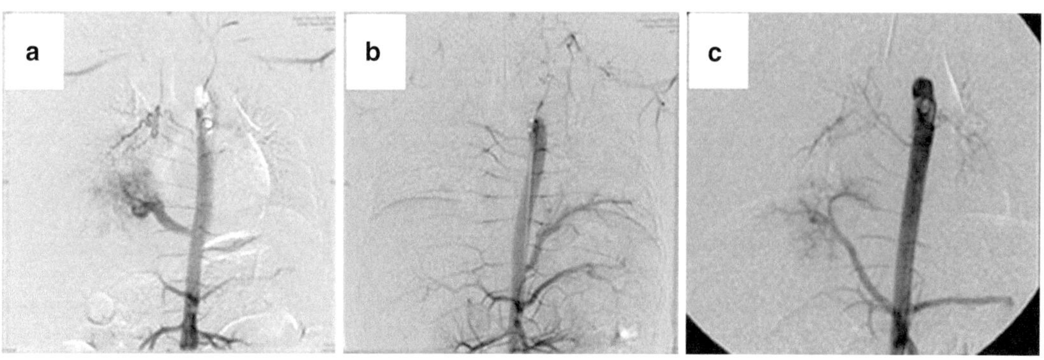


**Fig. 10.3** Aortic angiography to demonstrate aberrant arteries to the sequestered lung in ILS. (**a**) An aberrant artery branched from the thoracic aorta to the sequestered lung in the right lower lobe. (**b**) An aberrant artery branched from the abdominal aorta to the sequestered lung in the left lower lobe. (**c**) An aberrant artery branched from the celiac artery to the sequestered lung in the right lower lobe

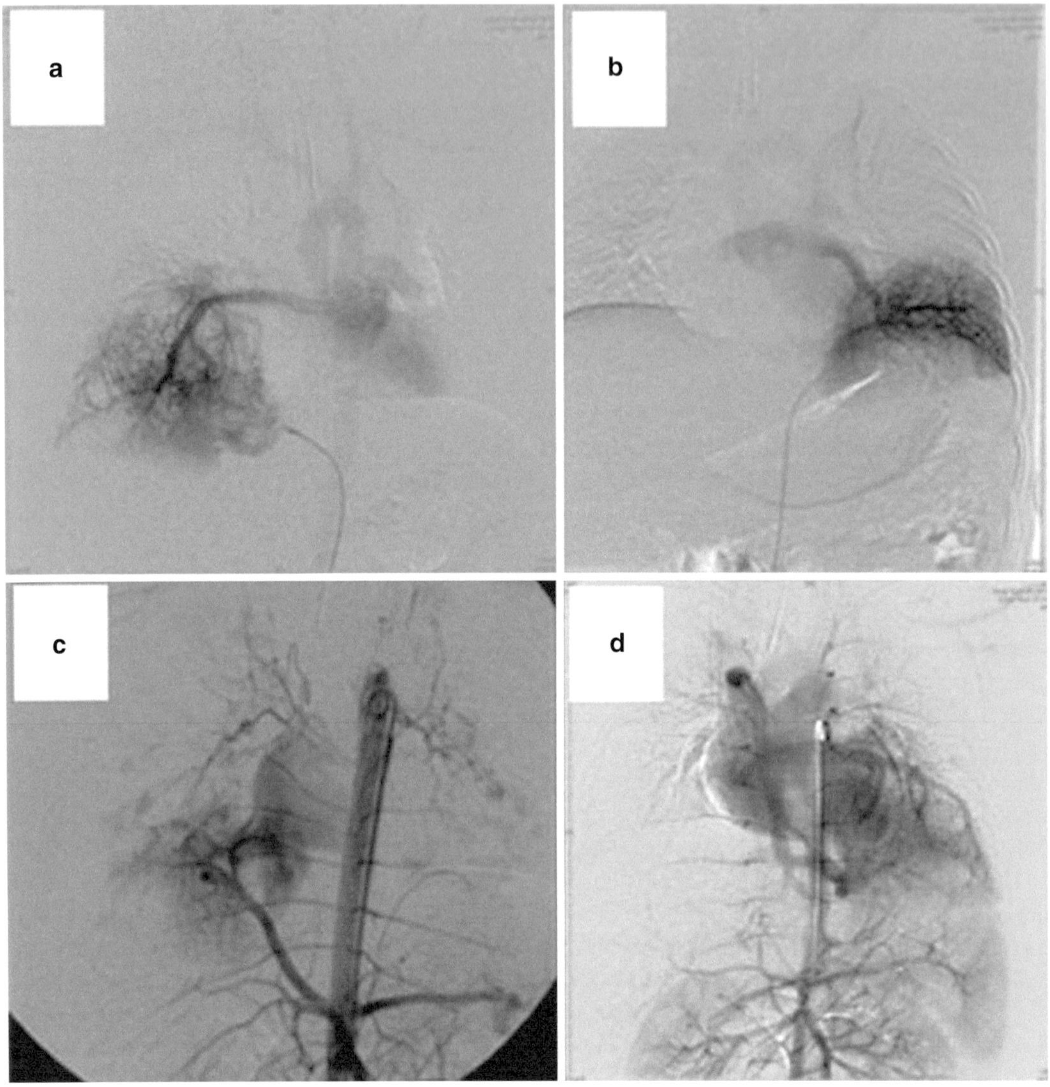


**Fig. 10.4** Representative cases of drainage veins from the sequestered lung. (**a**) The drainage vein from the sequestered lung is the left pulmonary vein as shown by selected angiography of the aberrant artery. (**b**) The drainage vein is the right pulmonary vein as shown by selected angiography of the aberrant artery. (**c**) The drainage vein is the inferior vena cava as shown by aortography. (**d**) The drainage veins are the azygos vein and left pulmonary vein as shown by aortography

aberrant artery feeds the lesion [27–32] (Fig. 10.2d) and each artery should be ligated separately to prevent unexpected bleeding. In two large case series [11, 12], the percentage of cases with more than one aberrant artery was 20.91% and 14.8%, respectively, and in our series it was 11.4% (4/35). The aberrant artery branched from the thoracic aorta (76.55% by Wei [11] and 73.9% by Savic [12]) or the abdominal aorta (18.47% by Wei [11] and 18.7% by Savic [12]) in the two previous case series. In our series, the aberrant artery branched from the thoracic aorta in 37.1% (Fig. 10.3a), the abdominal aorta in 48.6% (Fig. 10.3b) and the celiac artery in 14.3% (5/35) (Fig. 10.3c). Regarding the route of aberrant arteries, our data do not coincide with the data of large case series published in the past, but it is not clinically important because all aberrant arteries, whether they originated from the abdomen or thorax, were ligated in the thoracic cavity. In ILS, the drainage vein is the pulmonary vein in many cases (Fig. 10.4a, b). If the drainage vein connects to the systemic venous circulation (Fig. 10.4c, d), the drainage vein runs alongside the aberrant artery and unexpected venous damage may occur during the operation in such cases. The percentage of cases with systemic venous drainage was less than 10% among all ILS cases in the two large case series [11, 12], and it was 8.6% in our series, but we must always keep in mind that this rare venous return may exist in ILS.

## 10.6 Prognosis

The prognosis of ILS is satisfactory if appropriate lobectomy is performed after a correct diagnosis is made. Although ILS is a rare disease and it is difficult to obtain a correct diagnosis in some cases due to the nonspecific respiratory symptoms, it is important for physicians to suspect ILS and plan the correct imaging examination at the early stage.

## References

1. Pryce DM. Lower accessory pulmonary artery with intralobar sequestration of lung: a report of seven cases. J Pathol Bacteriol. 1946;58:457.
2. Takezoe T, Tahara K, Watanabe T, Ohno M, Kawasaki K, Higuchi M, Matsuo M, Nosaka S, Miyazaki O, Tsutsumi Y, Kanamori Y. Patterns of blood supply and venous drainage in pediatric intralobar pulmonary sequestration: a retrospective analysis of 30 pediatric cases from a single center. Open J Pediatr. 2016;6:274–9.
3. Genc O, Gurkok S, Dakak M, Gozubuyuk A, Ozakan M, Caylak H. Pulmonary sequestration and surgical treatment. Asian Cardiovasc Thorac Ann. 2006;14:3–6.
4. Kestenholz PB, Schneiter D, Hillinger S, Lardinois D, Weder W. Thoracoscopic treatment of pulmonary sequestration. Eur J Cardiothorac Surg. 2006;29:815–8.
5. Polaczek M, Baranska I, Szolkowska M, Zych J, Rudzinski P, Szopinski J, Orlowski T, Roszkowski-Sliz K. Clinical presentation and characteristics of 25 adult cases pulmonary sequestration. J Thoracic Dis. 2017;9:762–7.
6. Zhang N, Zeng Q, Chen C, Yu J, Zhang X. Distribution, diagnosis, and treatment of pulmonary sequestration: report of 208 cases. J Pediatr Surg. 2018;54: 1286–92.
7. Genç O, Gürkök S, Dakak M, Gözübüyük A, Özkan M, Çaylak H. Pulmonary sequestration and surgical treatment. Asian Cardiovasc Thorac Ann. 2006;14:3–6.
8. Marks C, Wiener SN, Reydman M. Pulmonary sequestration. Chest. 1972;61:253–7.
9. Buntain WL, Wooley MM, Mahour GH, Isaacs H Jr, Payne V Jr. Pulmonary sequestration in children: a twenty-five-year experience. Surgery. 1977;81:413–20.
10. Tashtoush B, Memarpour R, Gonzalez J, Gleason JB, Hadeh A. Pulmonary sequestration: a 29 patient case series and review. J Clin Diagn Res. 2015;9:5–8.
11. Wei Y, Li F. Pulmonary sequestration: a retrospective analysis of 2625 cases in China. Eur J Cardiothorac Surg. 2011;40:e39–42.
12. Savic B, Birtel FJ, Tholen W, Funke HD, Knoche R. Lung sequestration: report of seven cases and review of 540 published cases. Thorax. 1979;34:96–101.
13. Lim D, Kostin R. Intralobar pulmonary sequestration associated with Bochdalek hernia: first reported cases in an adult male and literature review. J Surg Case Rep. 2018;8:1–3.
14. Traibi A, Strauss C, Validire P, Gossot D. Intralobar pulmonary sequestration associated with bronchogenic cyst in adult. Asian Cardiovasc Thorac Ann. 2012;20:597–9.
15. Fumino S, Iwai N, Kimura O, Ono S, Higuchi K. Preoperative evaluation of the aberrant artery in intralobar pulmonary sequestration using multidetector computed tomography angiography. J Pediatr Surg. 2007;42:1776–9.
16. Wani SA, Mufti GN, Bhat NA, Baba AZ. Pulmonary sequestration: early diagnosis and management. Case Rep Pediatr. 2015;454860.
17. Qi W, Zhao J, Shi G, Yang F. Intralobar pulmonary sequestration displayed as localized emphysema on computed tomography image. J Cardiothorac Surg. 2017;12:83.
18. Mylan S, Maity S, Machlan J. Diagnosing intralobar pulmonary sequestration. Arch Dis Child. 2018;0:1.
19. Li K, Wu Q, Sun X, Geng Y, Leng D, Li H, Zhang S, Wang Q, Wu J, Xu L, Li X, Li Y, Zhang Q, Kurkciyan A, Liang J, Jiang D, Chen H. Tsp1 promotes alveolar stem cell proliferation and its down-regulation relates to lung inflammation in intralobar pulmonary sequestration. Oncotarget. 2017;39:64867–77.
20. Han P, Tian D, Yan W, Liu J, Chang Y, Xie W, Huang H. Pulmonary sequestration presenting with left upper abdominal bloating and marked elevation of serum carbohydrate antigen 19-9: a case report. Oncol Lett. 2014;7:1493–6.
21. Fu S, Wang H. Pulmonary sequestration associated with a synchronous elevation of carbohydrate antigen 50 and 19-9: a case report. Ann Transl Med. 2018;6:212.
22. Ahn SJ, Kim EY, Kim JH, Byun SS, Kim HS, Choi HY, Sun YH. Successful endovascular treatment of bilateral intralobar pulmonary sequestration with

a bridging isthmus in a child. Pediatr Pulmonol. 2014;49:E126–9.
23. Ojha V, Samui PP, Dakshit D. Role of endovascular embolization in improving the quality of life in a patient suffering from complicated intralobar pulmonary sequestration – a case report. Respir Med Case Rep. 2015;16:24–8.
24. Herbert CE, Reddy SRV, Lemler MS. Use of amplatzer vascular plugs for the treatment of combined extralobar and intralobar pulmonaru sequestration in a 5-year-old child. Cardiol Young. 2016;26:1441–4.
25. Ellis J, Brahmbhatt S, Desmond D, Ching B, Hostler J. Coil emobolization of intralobar pulmonary sequestration – an alternative to surgery: a case report. J Med Case Rep. 2018;12:375.
26. Yamanashi K, Okumura N, Nakazono C, Matsuoka T. Surgery for intralobar pulmonary sequestration using indocyanine green fluorescence navigation: a case report. Semin Thoracic Surg. 2018;30:122–4.
27. Jotsuka T, Matsuguma H, Sawafuji M, Yokoi K, Hirose K, Mori K, Tominaga Y, Imura J. Intralobar pulmonary sequestration with three aberrant arteries: a case report and review of the Japanese literature. Kyobu Geka. 1998;51:142–6.
28. Tsunezuka Y, Sato H. Intralobar pulmonary sequestration with three aberrant arteries in a 75-year-old patient. Chest. 1998;114:936–8.
29. Kanazawa S, Miyake T, Ishida A, Ohtani H, Tsunoda T, Tanemoto K. Intralobar pulmonary sequestration supplied by multiple anomalous arteries: report of a case. Surg Today. 2001;31:701–4.
30. Georgoff P, Singhal S. Multivessel intralobar pulmonary sequestration. Ann Thorac Sur. 2012;93:1318.
31. Theodoropoulos I, Schwartz MZ. Intralobar pulmonary sequestration: an uncommon case with triple arterial supply and systemic venous drainage. Pediatr Surg Int. 2012;28:741–4.
32. Erden ES, Yetim TD, Balci A, Akcay AB, Hakverdi S, Demirkose M. Intralobar pulmonary sequestration with arterial supply from two different origins: a case report. Ann Thorac Cardiovasc Surg. 2012;18: 560–3.

# 11 Surgical Treatment and Its Prognosis for Extra-lobar Pulmonary Sequestration Without Foregut Communication

Kyoko Mochizuki, Masato Shinkai, Norihiko Kitagawa, and Hidehito Usui

**Abstract**

Extra-lobar pulmonary sequestration (ELS) has a broad spectrum of clinical manifestations. When symptomatic, open or endoscopic sequestrectomy is indicated for its treatment with little objection. When asymptomatic, the natural course and appropriate treatment of ELS are controversial. In addition to surgery, transcatheter arterial embolization or continued observation is the therapeutic option for asymptomatic ELS. While surgery is curative in majority of patients, less invasive management is preferable, especially for asymptomatic ELS. Close and long-term follow-ups should be performed for patients who have avoided sequestrectomy.

**Keywords**

Extra-lobar pulmonary sequestration · Torsion · Treatment · Intrapericardial · Intraabdominal · Intradiaphragmatic · Endoscopic surgery · Prognosis

K. Mochizuki (✉) · M. Shinkai · N. Kitagawa
H. Usui
Department of Surgery, Kanagawa Children's Medical Center, Yokohama, Japan
e-mail: kmochizuki@kcmc.jp

## 11.1 Introduction

Extra-lobar pulmonary sequestration (ELS) accounts for 25% of all cases of pulmonary sequestrations [1, 2]. ELS is a congenital malformation characterized by cystic, nonfunctional embryonic lung tissue, which has no connection with the bronchial tree and receives its blood supply from the systemic circulation. It has a distinct pleural covering that is independent from that of the normal lungs [2–13]. The blood supply originates generally from the systemic circulation via the branches of the descending thoracic aorta or an aberrant branch of the abdominal aorta. The venous drainage usually flows into the systemic circulation via the azygos or portal veins [2, 6, 7, 10, 14].

Prenatal diagnosis of ELS is difficult, although it may account for up to 20% of prenatal pulmonary abnormalities. Without symptoms, sequestrations may go unrecognized for years [6, 15]. Around 60% of cases have associations with other abnormalities such as congenital diaphragmatic hernia, hydrops fetalis, and vertebral and cardiac malformations [7]. Incidentally, when detected, ELS must be differentiated from other mass-like lesions including neoplasms. ELS is occasionally symptomatic, even without other concomitant anomalies, because of infection, inflammation, hemorrhage, or infarction [2, 16].

The left hemithorax is the most commonly affected site, with reports of around 65% of ELS located between the left lower lobe and dia-


H. Sago et al. (eds.), *Congenital Cystic Lung Disease*, https://doi.org/10.1007/978-981-15-5175-8_11

phragm adjacent to the esophagus [1, 2, 7, 8, 14, 17, 18]. ELS has been reported to occur in the anterior mediastinum, upper thoracic region, and intrapericardial region and occasionally below the diaphragm [1, 2, 17]. Less than 10% of reported ELS cases occur outside the thorax [3], and 8% occur below the diaphragm [8].

ELS is usually asymptomatic in the prenatal period; during this time, some small lesions may undergo involution or disappear. However, a fetus with large lesions may develop ipsilateral pleural effusions, tension hydrothorax leading to hydrops fetalis, pulmonary hypoplasia, and pulmonary hypertension, which may require mechanical ventilation and possibly extracorporeal membrane oxygenation after delivery [9].

## 11.2 Location and Features of ELS

### 11.2.1 Torsion

The vascular pedicles of ELS rarely undergo torsion resulting in infarction [19–22]. Infarcted ELS manifests with chest or abdominal pain [2]. ELS complicated by hemorrhagic infarction is generally diagnosed based on the following imaging findings: (1) Polygonadal mass in the paravertebral region, (2) a homogeneous high-density mass enhancing only on the periphery on computed tomography (CT), (3) reactive pleural effusion or hemothorax, and (4) no feeding artery identified. Lack of enhancement in the peripheral portion of the lesion and internal hemorrhage are important clues suggesting hemorrhagic infarction [2, 19]. Inflammatory markers including C-reactive protein may be elevated. Chest X-ray findings in patients with torsion of ELS are nonspecific, with lower lobar opacity and/or pleural effusion. Ultrasonography shows a well-circumscribed echogenic mass, without vascularity or a feeding vessel. CT and/or magnetic resonance imaging (MRI) likewise, show a well-defined, ovoid mass without an identifiable feeding vessel (Fig. 11.1a, b). Pathologically, torsion of ELS is characterized by hemorrhagic coagulative necrosis with residual identifiable lung architecture [21]. While urgent sequestrectomy should be performed for torsion causing respiratory distress due to pleural effusion or hemothorax, patients without respiratory distress may be observed without treatment, because ELS after torsion may regress spontaneously.

### 11.2.2 Intrapericardial ELS

Intrapericardial ELS has seldom been described [23]. Based on case reports, intrapericardial ELS can be misdiagnosed preoperatively as intraperi-

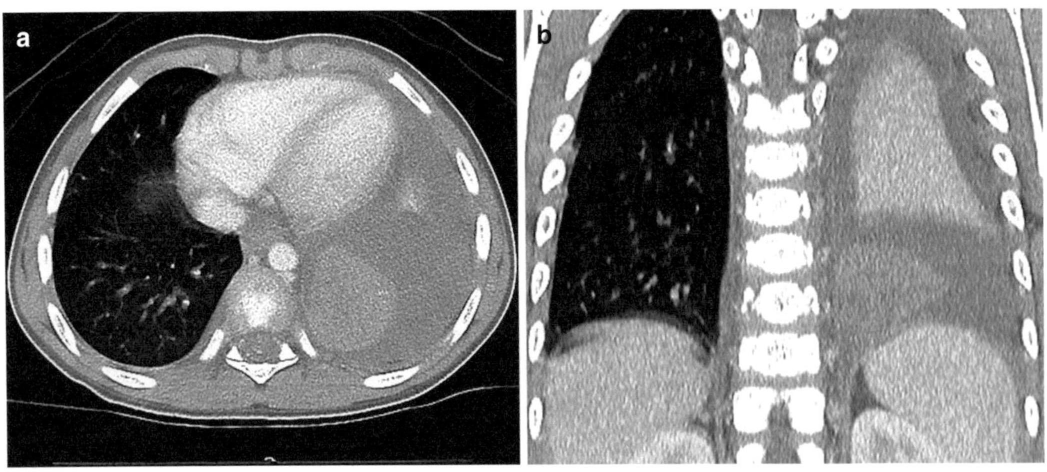


**Fig. 11.1** Torsion of vascular pedicles of ELS; a well-defined, ovoid mass without an identifiable feeding vessel on: (**a**) Cross-sectional imaging with CT and (**b**) Frontal-sectional imaging with CT

cardial teratoma [24]. Symptoms include pericardial effusion, cardiac tamponade, tachypnea, pneumothorax, tachycardia, and dyspnea [24, 25]. Aberrant arteries feeding the intrapericardial ELS originate from various arteries, including the innominate artery, subclavian artery, and pulmonary artery. Early resection has been recommended for two reasons: first, to obtain a precise diagnosis; and second, to prevent cardiac failure. In intrapericardial teratoma, which is reported frequently, 48.5% of patients have prenatal cardiac tamponade and hydrops fetalis. Therefore, intrapericardial ELS, similar to intrapericardial teratoma, requires close monitoring for cardiac failure, and early resection has been undertaken frequently during the neonatal period and lead to good prognosis [24, 25].

### 11.2.3 Intraabdominal ELS

An intraabdominal ELS, fed by the abdominal aorta, is usually stable and rarely grows aggressively. Intraabdominal ELS rarely causes high-output cardiac failure or interrupts venous return because most lesions are located on the left side, far away from the inferior vena cava [3]. The treatment of intraabdominal ELS is controversial. The natural course and consequences of intraabdominal ELS are still not well known. Because intraabdominal ELS is usually asymptomatic with exceptionally rare complications such as malignancy or infection [3, 8] and spontaneous regression is likely, conservative management has been advocated. However, surgical resection remains the principal treatment, because complete excision can confirm the diagnosis by histopathological analysis [8], and postsurgical (both open and endoscopic) outcomes of isolated intraabdominal ELS have been satisfactory [3].

### 11.2.4 Intradiaphragmatic ELS

Intradiaphragmatic ELS is extremely rare [14, 18, 26]. Because of its unique location, it is necessary to rule out neuroblastoma, adrenal hematoma, or teratoma [26]. Imaging for diagnosis of intradiaphragmatic ELS is not easy [18]. After birth, coronal reformatted images from contrast-enhanced CT might show the split hemidiaphragm sign, which demonstrates two identifiable leaflets of the diaphragmatic muscle encasing the mass, suggestive of intradiaphragmatic localization [14, 18, 27]. Some intradiaphragmatic lesions have also been found incidentally during diaphragmatic hernia surgery [17].

In some reports, the thoracic approach for diaphragmatic ELS is recommended, and the abdominal approach is adopted only when the preoperative diagnosis is intraabdominal ELS [17, 18, 26, 27]. However, because preoperative imaging studies cannot always differentiate whether a sequestration is intraabdominal, intrathoracic, or intradiaphragmatic, operative planning may pose a challenge. Recently, a combination of two surgical approaches has been recommended: single-cavity and dual-cavity exploration, with a combined thoracoscopic and laparoscopic approach. The use of minimally invasive approaches can allow exploration of both, the thoracic and abdominal cavities with low morbidity [10, 14, 28].

## 11.3 Treatment

### 11.3.1 Indications

#### 11.3.1.1 Symptomatic ELS

Surgery should be considered for patients with symptomatic ELS causing recurrent pulmonary infection, hemorrhage, gastrointestinal symptoms, or heart failure. In neonates, surgery is indicated when the mass increases in size, and urgent action is needed in case of respiratory distress [12, 15, 29] associated with massive pleural effusion (Fig. 11.2a–d) [15, 30].

#### 11.3.1.2 Asymptomatic ELS

There are several treatment options for patients with asymptomatic ELS, including surgical resection, transcatheter arterial embolization (TAE), and observation without treatment. Reportedly, ELS can show spontaneous regression without treatment, and there have been few

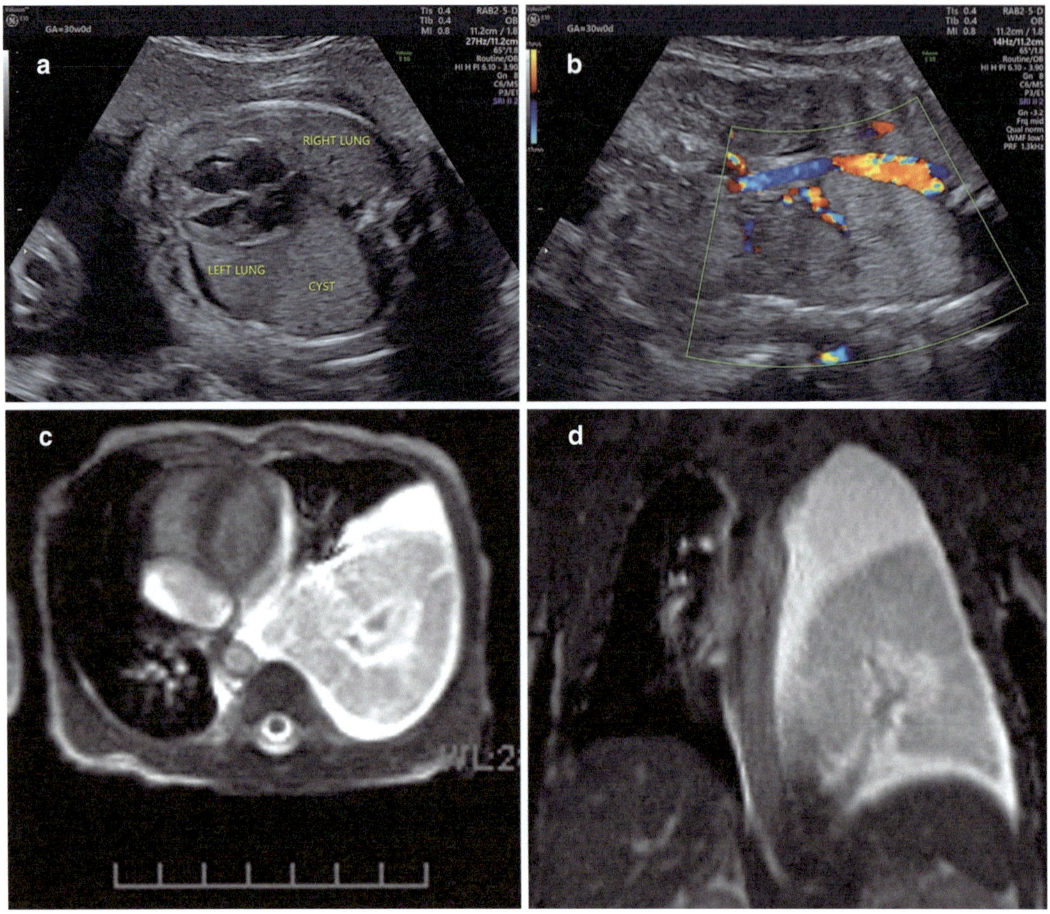


**Fig. 11.2** Large lesions are associated with the development of ipsilateral pleural effusions. (**a**) Prenatal thoracic mass on ultrasonography, (**b**) Prenatal blood supply for thoracic mass on ultrasonography, (**c**) and (**d**) Ipsilateral pleural effusions with large mass lesions

reports of malignant transformation [10, 15, 18, 20, 27, 30–33]. However, because the natural course of asymptomatic ELS is not completely understood, no management guidelines have been established for children with incidentally diagnosed ELS, nor is there consensus about the appropriate timing for surgery [13, 15, 23]. Considering the possible risk of infection and malignant transformation, preemptive surgical treatment may be advisable [15], although surgery or TAE may pose a potential risk of surgical complications in young patients [32]. Once ELS is complicated by torsion or infection, subsequent edema or pleural adhesion makes the surgery difficult and increases the risk of postoperative bleeding, infection, pneumothorax, and poor healing [15, 33].

### 11.3.2 Surgery

Surgery is usually justified because the definitive diagnosis depends on histopathological examination [12, 29]. The surgical treatment of choice is sequestrectomy, in which the vascular pedicle is carefully ligated and divided (Fig. 11.3a–d) [1, 6, 20]. Massive hemorrhage has been reported to occur during adhesiolysis [15] or when the feeding arteries are missing or improperly ligated [1, 6, 34]. Sequestrectomy can be performed through open thoracotomy or video-assisted thoracic surgery (VATS) approach [5]. Although postoperative morbidity may be reduced by minimally invasive techniques, indication for resection should be individualized on the basis of the patient's lesion, health status, and family wishes [12, 13, 28, 29, 33].

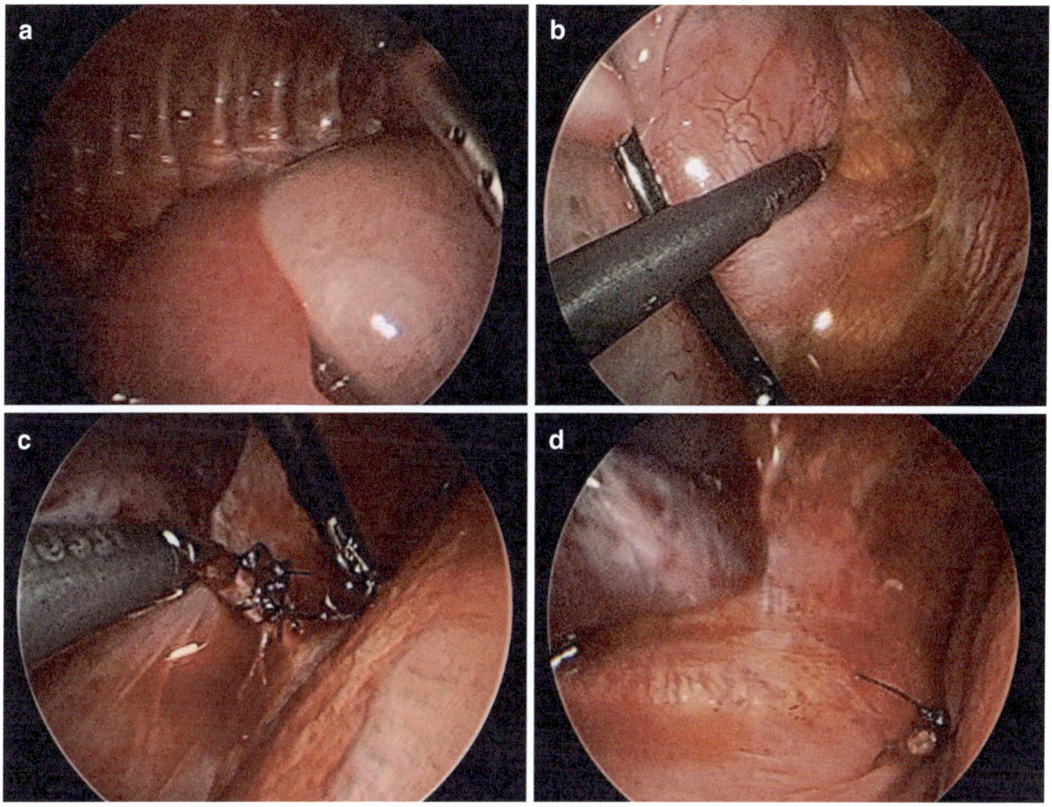


**Fig. 11.3** Thoracoscopic sequestrectomy. (**a**) Thoracoscopic view of ELS, (**b**) Vascular pedicle of ELS, (**c**) Ligation of the vascular pedicle, (**d**) Dissection of the vascular pedicle

#### 11.3.2.1 Thoracotomy

Surgery is usually performed through posterolateral thoracotomy or laparotomy [11, 12]. Recently, thoracotomy using axillary incision with muscle sparing has been performed often for the prevention of thoracic deformity after surgery.

#### 11.3.2.2 Endoscopic Surgery

VATS, thoracoscopic surgery, and laparoscopic surgery require minimal incisions, resulting in lesser postoperative pain, smaller esthetic scars, and faster recovery [11, 12]. All the procedures begin with occlusion of feeding vessels by ligation, clipping, sealing (LigaSure™ bipolar cautery), or stapling [4, 12, 16]. There may be multiple aberrant arteries [4]. The magnified view of the operative field provided by endoscopy is particularly useful in detecting small vessels, such as feeding arteries and drainage veins [1]. Minimally invasive surgery using endoscopic techniques with magnification lenses allows easier visualization and separation of the interface between tissues during surgery [26].

##### VATS/Thoracoscopic Surgery

VATS procedure has been shown to be safe and to have a low rate of postoperative complications [6, 20]. Under single-lung ventilation, the patient is placed in the lateral decubitus position supported by an air pillow, and the upper extremities are extended forward [4]. Three or five ports are needed to perform the resection. The trocars are placed on the anterior, middle, and posterior axillary lines between the fourth and the eighth intercostal spaces to obtain a good manipulation angle for active instrument ports [16]. After removing intrathoracic adhesions and identifying aberrant vessels, the abnormal artery is dissected at a point closest to the lung tissue to secure enough length to ligate and divide the vessel safely [4]. Thoracoscopy provides a wider view of exposure by the 30-degree lenses, especially when the adhesion being treated is between the lung and the diaphragm surface or at the cardiophrenic angle. Magnified surgical fields by thoracoscopy help to identify the boundaries between lung tissue and inflammatory scars. VATS should be performed by experienced surgeons because of the potential risk of life-threatening vascular injury [4]. The thoracoscopic approach yields a superior cosmetic result and reduces the risk of scoliosis and chest-wall deformity. The postoperative stay seems to be shorter with this procedure than with the conventional technique, but these findings need to be confirmed in a prospective and more detailed study [16].

**Laparoscopic Surgery**

Laparoscopic resection for intraabdominal ELS is safe and effective, but careful preoperative imaging studies are recommended to plan the most suitable approach [35]. The intraabdominal approach allows good visualization and precise control of the feeding vessels arising from the abdominal segment of the aorta. Retroesophageal laparoscopic dissection allows an excellent view of the mass and safe control of the systemic feeding vessels [12]. The laparoscopic procedure is performed in the supine decubitus position. A Hasson trocar is placed in the umbilicus. Under direct vision, three or five ports are necessary to perform the resection. After the ELS is detached, the specimen is removed through the umbilical incision [12].

### 11.3.3 TAE

Some reports have suggested the noninvasive endovascular approach (Amplatzer™ occlusive devices and coils to exclude the inflow of the aberrant vessels) as an exclusive (alternative to surgery) therapeutic option in selected cases of pulmonary sequestration [20, 36]. Embolization of the feeding systemic artery is a valuable presurgery procedure or alternative to surgery. However, TAE is a challenging treatment for pediatric and interventional cardiologists and careful analysis of procedural results and its benefits at long-term follow-up are necessary because TAE alone cannot excise the lesion in its entirety [27, 29, 31].

To assess the presence of residual pulmonary sequestration including of vascularization is required for follow-up of regression of pulmonary sequestration tissue after TAE. MRI is more appropriate to study pulmonary sequestration parenchyma and vascularization (enhancement) than thorax CT, which would expose infants to high dose of radiations [31].

### 11.3.4 Conservative Management

Conservative management and long-term follow-up have also been recommended because of the possibility of disappearance or spontaneous regression. However, conservative management is inevitably accompanied by the lack of pathological confirmation of the lesion, which leads to a stressful long-term follow-up. Natural history and long-term sequelae of ELS are unknown, while pathological features of ELS that comprise both elements of pulmonary sequestration and congenital pulmonary airway malformation may suggest a higher malignant potential of ELS than is generally presumed [12, 13, 28, 29, 33].

## 11.4 Prognosis

Pulmonary sequestration has very low morbidity and excellent long-term outcome [37]. It is generally well known that ELS can spontaneously regress; however, the exact mechanism remains unclear [32]. For the management of asymptomatic ELS, the risks of surgical morbidity must be weighed against the risks of complications of the ELS itself, such as repeated infections [1]. Various complications including infection with recurrent pneumonia, hemothorax, torsion with/without infarction, high-output heart failure due to the left to right shunt, or malignancy have been reported in the literature. However, these complications are quite rare in clinical practice [33]. Patients who did not undergo surgical treatment after birth should be followed up for a long time [15, 33]. Although malignancy arising from pulmonary sequestrations is rare, adenocarcinoma arising secondary to ELS has been reported. The etiology of the carcinomas in the sequestration cases may be multifactorial and may include chronic inflammation and irritation [33].

## 11.5 Conclusion

Sequestrectomy is an effective treatment for symptomatic ELS including torsion. Endoscopic surgery should be performed by experienced surgeons. The clinical course and treatment of asymptomatic ELS are controversial. Although the surgical outcome is satisfactory in majority of the patients, less invasive management for asymptomatic ELS needs to be established. Close and long-term follow-ups should be performed for patients who have not undergone sequestrectomy.

**Acknowledgment** The authors wish to acknowledge Dr. Kawataki, Department of Neonatology, for his help with prenatal diagnosis.

## References

1. Fukui T, Hakiri S, Yokoi K. Extralobar pulmonary sequestration in the middle mediastinum. Gen Thorac Cardiovasc Surg. 2017;65(8):481–3.
2. Takeuchi K, et al. Two adult cases of extralobar pulmonary sequestration: a non-complicated case and a necrotic case with torsion. Pol J Radiol. 2014;79:145–9.
3. Xu G, et al. Prenatal diagnosis of fetal intraabdominal extralobar pulmonary sequestration: a 12-year 3-center experience in China. Sci Rep. 2019;9(1):943.
4. Wang S, Li Y, Wang J. Video-assisted thoracoscopic surgery for pulmonary sequestrations: series of 35 consecutive patients in a single center. Thorac Cardiovasc Surg. 2019;67(1):73–8.
5. Dell'Amore A, et al. Uniportal thoracoscopic resection of intralobar and extralobar pulmonary sequestration. J Vis Surg. 2018;4:63.
6. Greenspon A, Samuels L, Greenspon L. Extralobar sequestration complicated by a cystic hamartoma in an adult. Ann Thorac Surg. 2018;108:e43–4.
7. Pires CR, et al. Diagnosis of intra-abdominal extralobar pulmonary sequestration by means of ultrasound in a neonate. Case Rep Pediatr. 2013;2013:623102.
8. Costa MR, et al. Atypical presentation of intra-abdominal extralobar pulmonary sequestration detected in prenatal care: a case report. Rev Paul Pediatr. 2016;34(2):243–6.
9. Mychaliska GB, et al. Giant pulmonary sequestration: the rare case requiring the EXIT procedure with resection and ECMO. Fetal Diagn Ther. 2009;25(1):163–6.
10. Escobar MA Jr, Acierno SP. Laparoscopic resection of an intradiaphragmatic pulmonary sequestration: a case report and review of the literature. J Pediatr Surg. 2012;47(11):2129–33.
11. Tamura M, Shimizu Y, Hashizume Y. Single-incision video-assisted thoracic resection for extrapulmonary sequestration: a case report. J Cardiothorac Surg. 2014;9:22.
12. Joyeux L, et al. Ectopic extralobar pulmonary sequestrations in children: interest of the laparoscopic approach. J Pediatr Surg. 2010;45(11):2269–73.
13. Alsumrain M, Ryu JH. Pulmonary sequestration in adults: a retrospective review of resected and unresected cases. BMC Pulm Med. 2018;18(1):97.
14. Alamo L, Gudinchet F, Meuli R. Imaging findings in fetal diaphragmatic abnormalities. Pediatr Radiol. 2015;45(13):1887–900.
15. Hong C, et al. Risk analysis and outcomes of bronchopulmonary sequestrations. Pediatr Surg Int. 2017;33(9):971–5.
16. Bonnard A, et al. Pulmonary sequestration children: is the thoracoscopic approach a good option? Surg Endosc. 2004;18(9):1364–7.
17. Zhang N, et al. Distribution, diagnosis, and treatment of pulmonary sequestration: report of 208 cases. J Pediatr Surg. 2018;54:1286–92.
18. Lee JH, Kim MJ. Intradiaphragmatic extralobar pulmonary sequestration in adult. J Cardiothorac Surg. 2014;9:112.
19. Choe J, Goo HW. Extralobar pulmonary sequestration with hemorrhagic infarction in a child: preoperative imaging diagnosis and pathological correlation. Korean J Radiol. 2015;16(3):662–7.
20. Houda el M, et al. Antenatal diagnosis of extralobar pulmonary sequestration. Pan Afr Med J. 2014;19:54.
21. Zucker EJ, et al. Paediatric torsed extralobar sequestration containing calcification: imaging findings with pathological correlation. Clin Radiol. 2013;68(1):94–7.
22. Chen W, et al. Extralobar pulmonary sequestration presenting with torsion: a case report and review of literature. J Pediatr Surg. 2011;46(10):2025–8.
23. Wei Y, et al. Intrapericardial extralobar pulmonary sequestration in adult. Ann Thorac Surg. 2013;95(3):1093–6.
24. Yanagisawa S, et al. Intrapericardial extralobar pulmonary sequestration detected as an intrathoracic cystic mass by using prenatal ultrasonography: case report and review of the literature. J Pediatr Surg. 2012;47(12):2327–31.
25. de Vreede I, et al. Intrapericardial extralobar pulmonary sequestration presenting as a prenatal intrathoracic mass. Pediatr Cardiol. 2008;29(5):980–2.

26. Chun H, et al. Diagnosis and management of intradiaphragmatic extralobar pulmonary sequestration: a report of 11 cases. J Pediatr Surg. 2015;50(8):1269–72.
27. Meier AH, Eggli KD, Cilley RE. Intradiaphragmatic extralobar sequestration-a rare pulmonary anomaly. J Pediatr Surg. 2009;44(12):e27–9.
28. Nijagal A, et al. The diagnosis and management of intradiaphragmatic extralobar pulmonary sequestrations: a report of 4 cases. J Pediatr Surg. 2012;47(8):1501–5.
29. Ballouhey Q, et al. Pulmonary and intestinal congenital anomalies masquerading as cystic suprarenal masses. Eur J Pediatr Surg. 2012;22(6):434–8.
30. Divjak N, et al. Bronchopulmonary sequestration with morbid neonatal pleural effusion despite successful antenatal treatment. Front Pediatr. 2017;5:259.
31. Borgia F, et al. Clinical benefits, echocardiographic and MRI assessment after pulmonary sequestration treatment. Int J Cardiol. 2017;240:165–71.
32. Yoon HM, et al. Extralobar pulmonary sequestration in neonates: the natural course and predictive factors associated with spontaneous regression. Eur Radiol. 2017;27(6):2489–96.
33. Belchis D, et al. Adenocarcinoma arising in an extralobar sequestration: a case report and review of the literature. Lung Cancer. 2014;84(1):92–5.
34. Shadmehr MB, et al. Extralobar sequestration in anterior mediastinum with pericardial agenesis. Ann Thorac Surg. 2009;88(1):291–3.
35. Moreno-Sanz C, et al. Intra-abdominal pulmonary secuestration as an exceptional cause of abdominal mass in the adult. Int J Surg Case Rep. 2013;4(11):997–9.
36. Mengoli MC, et al. Malignant pigmented mass "sequestrated" in the lung: a unique case report. Lung. 2016;194(4):699–701.
37. Chong NV, Polley TZ Jr, Geiger JD. Infarction of extralobar pulmonary sequestration after blunt trauma. J Pediatr Surg. 2007;42(6):1127–9.

# 12 Surgical Treatment and Its Prognosis for Extralobar Pulmonary Sequestration with Foregut Communication: Communicating Bronchopulmonary Foregut Malformation (CBPFM)

Kosaku Maeda

**Abstract**

In 1968, Gerle introduced the term "bronchopulmonary foregut malformation (BPFM)" in connection with pulmonary sequestration with a communication with the esophagus or stomach. BPFM has recently been proposed to apply to all abnormalities of the tracheobronchial tree originating during development from the foregut. Communicating bronchopulmonary foregut malformation (CBPFM) is defined by congenital communication between the esophagus or stomach and an isolated part of the airway.

For the treatment of this type of complex foregut anomaly, arriving at a correct diagnosis is the most important factor in determining the appropriate operative management. There are able to sort out the anatomy by radiologic imaging and bronchoscopy.

The affected respiratory system is often resected because it is usually not working when diagnosed because of severe pneumonia or hypoplasia or agenesis itself. According to the Srikant category, CBPFM Group IA was difficult to diagnose, had a high mortality rate. Pneumonectomy was performed in most patients with group IA or group II. In early infancy, total pneumonectomy induces asymmetric growth of the chest, which can lead to risk of postpneumonectomy syndrome as the patient grows. There should be performed serial operations to successfully preserve the affected lung, air way, and reconstruct the esophagus.

**Keywords**

Communicating bronchopulmonary foregut malformation · Extralobar sequestration Esophageal lung

## 12.1 Introduction

Pulmonary sequestration is a congenital malformation within the spectrum of bronchopulmonary foregut malformations. This pathological condition was first described by Rokitansky [1] and Rektorzik [2] in 1861 by the term "accessory lobe." It was renamed "pulmonary sequestration" by Price [3] in 1946.

K. Maeda (✉)
Department of Pediatric Surgery,
Kobe Children's Hospital, Kobe, Japan



H. Sago et al. (eds.), *Congenital Cystic Lung Disease*, https://doi.org/10.1007/978-981-15-5175-8_12

This type of malformation of the lung receives blood supply from one or more systemic arteries and may or may not communicate with the bronchial tree. The incidence of pulmonary sequestration ranges from 0.15% to 1.7% [4]. Two different forms are described: intralobar and extralobar. Extralobar sequestration is completely isolated from the lungs and usually has its own pleural covering. Infradiaphragmatic pulmonary sequestration belongs to the extralobar type, and most cases have been reported in the suprarenal region associated with other congenital malformations [5].

In 1968, Gerle et al. [6] introduced the term "bronchopulmonary foregut malformation" in connection with pulmonary sequestration with a communication with the esophagus or stomach. The name "bronchopulmonary foregut malformation" has recently been proposed to apply to all abnormalities of the tracheobronchial tree originating during development from the foregut [8].

## 12.2 Definition

Bronchopulmonary foregut malformations include a wide spectrum of airway anomalies that occur due to abnormal separation of the primitive foregut and esophagus. The spectrum includes four main types: foregut anomalies, vascular abnormalities, lung parenchymal abnormalities, and airway anomalies. Each type has its own pathology and presentations. Examples of these anomalies include congenital pulmonary airway malformations (CPAM), bronchogenic cysts, pulmonary sequestration, congenital lobar emphysema, esophageal atresia with or without tracheoesophageal fistula, and bronchial atresia or stenosis. There may be overlap between these anomalies (hybrid lesions), and multiple pathologies coexist in the same lesion [15].

Communicating bronchopulmonary foregut malformation (CBPFM) is a rare congenital anomaly defined by congenital communication between the esophagus or stomach and an isolated part of the airway. Lesions associated with the pulmonary lobe bronchus originating from the esophagus are called esophageal bronchi. When the main bronchus comes from the esophagus, it is called the esophageal lung [16]. Gerle et al. [6] introduced the term CBPFM to describe cases of pulmonary sequestration with patent communication to the gastrointestinal tract. Affected lungs often receive a systemic blood supply [9]. CBPFM occurs when there is congenital communication between the lung and the foregut due to a focal mesoderm defect [6, 16].

When the primitive main bronchus is attached to the esophagus, the anomaly is known as the "esophageal lung" [6]. The esophageal lung was first described by Keeley et al. in 1960 [10] and is considered a rare type of extralobar sequestration. Other congenital anomalies can coexist in association with the esophageal lung. For example, esophageal lung with esophageal atresia and tracheoesophageal fistula has been reported in about half of reported cases [6, 11, 12]. Other related symptoms such as duodenal atresia, duodenal stenosis, and congenital heart disease have been reported [13, 14].

Srikanth et al. [8] devised a system that can classify CBPFM into four main groups. Group I is associated with esophageal atresia and tracheoesophageal fistula, with two subdivisions: group IA in which the main bronchus is absent, and the entire lung originates from the esophagus or stomach, and group IB contains only a portion of one lung that is communicating with the esophagus. Group II features are the absence of the main bronchus arising from the trachea and the presence of one hypoplastic lung (usually right) arising from the esophagus. Group III occurs when an isolated part of the lungs communicates with the esophagus, and Group IV occurs when the normal bronchial system communicates with the esophagus (Fig. 12.1).

## 12.3 Epidemiology

Clinical symptoms depend on the type of abnormality, the site of communication, and the associated anomalies. Most cases appear early in life, but there is one report that appears late at age of 20 years [14]. Early diagnosis of CBPFM is dif-

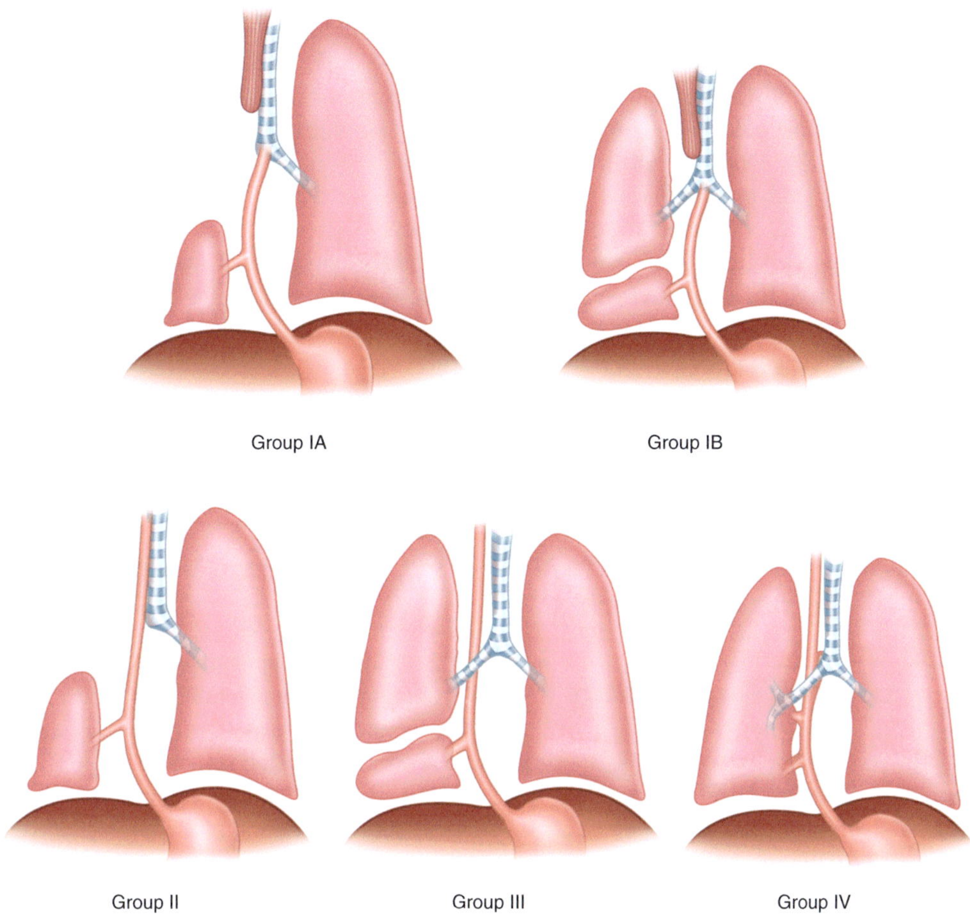


**Fig. 12.1** Classification of CBPFM (From reference [8]. Srikanth MS, Ford EG, Stanley P, Mahour GH. Communicating bronchopulmonary foregut malformations: classification and embryogenesis. J Pediatr Surg. 1992; 27:732–6)

ficult due to the rare and nonspecific symptoms of this entity.

### 12.3.1 Classification and Affected Side [7]

Of the 61 cases included, 13 cases in Group IA (21.3%), 4 cases in Group IB (6.6%), 18 cases in Group II (29.5%), 23 cases in Group III (37.7%), and 3 cases (4.9%) were Group IV cases [7]. Most malformations were on the right (72.1 vs. 23.0%). 3.3% had bilateral malformations. The left/right ratio was 3.1:1. Abnormal lung tissue blood supply was reported in 39 cases, 17 cases from the pulmonary artery and 22 cases from the systemic artery.

### 12.3.2 Gestation and Family History [7]

Polyhydramnios was reported in 10 cases (3 in Group I, 3 in Group II, 3 in Group III, and 1 in Group IV) [7]. Fetal MRI detected tubular structures toward the gastroesophageal junction during the fifth trimester of pregnancy. These five cases belonged to group III. In two cases, a mass was detected in the fetal thoracic cavity.

## 12.4 Pathogenesis

The embryologic basis for the development of CBPFM and other congenital anomalies of the lower airway is not fully understood. The most widely accepted embryological theory is that BPFM occurs early in the pseudo glandular stage of pulmonary development (5–17 weeks of gestation) prior to the separation of the aorta and pulmonary circulation. This is the widespread observed, including the connection to the systemic circulation, the presence of a separate visceral pleura in extralobar sequestration, or its lack in intralobar sequestration. These characteristics explain the pathology of congenital pulmonary airway malformations (CPAM), occasional association with bronchogenic cysts or connection to the foregut, and related abnormalities such as congenital diaphragmatic hernia.

## 12.5 Anatomical Characteristics

Sequestrations are characterized by its location, connection to the lungs or other structures, vascular supply, and association with other abnormalities. By definition, arterial blood supply comes from the systemic circulation.

Associated malformations [7]: Because CBPFM Group I is related to esophageal closure and tracheoesophageal fistula (EA/TEF), EA/TEF is not included as a related malformation. Cardiovascular abnormalities are the most common associated malformations (18.0%), followed by VACTERL-association (9.8%), skeletal malformations (9.8%), anorectal malformations (3.3%), diaphragmatic hernia (3.3%), and other rare malformations.

## 12.6 Clinical Findings and Symptoms

In the majority of cases, the lesion regresses during the course of gestation. Occasionally, hydrops develops, likely because of vascular compression. There are no reliable criteria for determining which lesions will grow and develop hydrops versus those that will stabilize or regress.

Most initial symptoms range from asymptomatic to fatal, including recurrent aspiration and collapse of the affected lung. If CBPFM is associated with long-segment congenital tracheal stenosis, a mortality rate of 28% has been reported [18].

Twenty patients had dyspnea after birth [7]. Group I patients showed drooling, feeding intolerance, and nasogastric tube failure due to esophageal atresia. Recurrent respiratory infections with cough and fever were the main symptoms in older children and adults (45.5%). Other symptoms include cough/suffocation after food intake, hemoptysis, nocturnal cough, and epigastric pain.

### 12.6.1 Evaluation and Diagnosis

Based on prenatal ultrasonography, extralobar sequestration may be initially suspected. Later, if an abnormal systemic artery can be identified with confidence, a temporary diagnosis can be made with advanced imaging (CT or MRI).

Prenatal diagnosis is difficult and is most often diagnosed during histopathological studies of resected masses found by routine ultrasonography. The final definitive diagnosis is made only by pathological examination after surgical resection.

A number of ultrasonographic features are described to help with differential diagnosis, such as the presence of calcification in a homogeneous, echogenic mass. Differential diagnosis includes suprarenal neuroblastoma, teratomas, foregut duplication, and CPFM. The latter is also a congenital lung anomaly characterized by a mass of cysts that may contain different types of tissues such as cartilage, muscle, and mucous glands.

Diagnosis is usually made during a radiological examination of persistent or recurrent lung collapse despite ventilatory support (Fig. 12.2). CT can easily identify the absence of the main bronchus arising from the trachea and can be used to assess the location of anomalous airway. The use of intravenous contrast medium may identify associated thoracic and extrathoracic

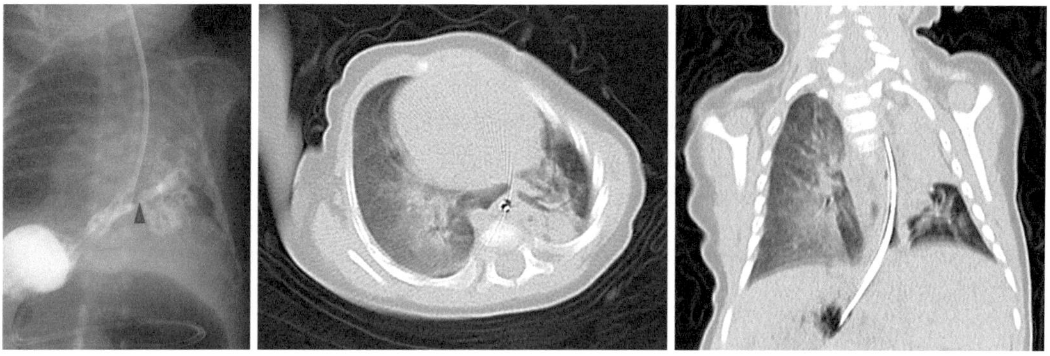

**Fig. 12.2** Esophagogram and chest CT in Group II patient. The communication with the esophagus is shown (arrow)

vascular anomalies. Upper gastrointestinal contrast studies using oral water-soluble contrast medium is the golden standard method for identifying the abnormal origin of the airway from the esophagus and identifying the condition of the remaining esophagus. MRI of surgically proven esophageal bronchus was able to identify a bronchial abnormality in the form of a T2-hyperintense tubular structure directed from the lung to the gastroesophageal junction in the prenatal period [19].

In group I, chest radiographs were obtained at 70.6% [7]. A vague half-chest and right ventricular mediastinal shift of 52.9% and 17.6% was found in low or normal lungs. 82.4% of Group I CBPFM were misdiagnosed and underwent surgery for EA/TEF (mainly esophageal anastomosis or stomach or construction ligation). A definitive diagnosis was confirmed by further assessment promoted by persistent atelectasis of one lung, refractory dyspnea, or routine postoperative UGI. Ipsilateral lung opacification and mediastinal shift were also uniform symptoms of group II (100%) chest radiographs. Group III and group IV plain X-rays were reported at 42.3%. Symptoms varied, including mediastinal or lung mass (19.2%) and partial stiffness of the lung (23.1%).

The diagnosis of CBPFM was confirmed by UGI (62.3%), CT (11.5%), bronchoscopy (1.6%), and intraoperative findings (13.1%) [7]. There were five cases (8.2%) diagnosed by ultrasonography and fetal MRI before birth.

## 12.7 Treatment

Treatment of intra-abdominal pulmonary sequestration is controversial. Spontaneous regression has been reported in 12 patients; some authors have suggested close follow-up with imaging. However, if a diagnosis of neuroblastoma or cystic adenoma malformation cannot be ruled out, surgical resection must be performed [20].

In the literature, approximately 140 CBPFM cases have been reported [21]. The affected respiratory system is often resected because it is usually not working when diagnosed because of severe pneumonia or hypoplasia or agenesis itself. According to the Srikant category, CBPFM Group IA was difficult to diagnose, had a high mortality rate, and no one survived preservation of affected lungs [8]. Pneumonectomy was performed in most patients with group IA or group II. Unilateral lung resection in neonates and infants was well tolerated. However, the prevalence of long-term consequences, such as chest wall deformation, scoliosis, and postpneumonectomy syndrome were unclear. In early infancy, total pneumonectomy induces asymmetric growth of the chest, which can lead to risk of postpneumonectomy syndrome as the patient grows [24].

Some authors described efforts to reconstruct the bronchi with CBPFM [9–12, 15], but mortality was high. Attempts have been made to reconstruct tracheobronchial CBPFM to preserve the affected lungs [22, 23], but the first successful tracheobronchial reconstruction of CBPFM is awaited until 1997. Michel et al. [17] reported for the first time that esophageal bronchial reconstruction was successful in CBPFM group II of two patients. They concluded that the lungs with abnormal circulation need to be removed. Reconstruction of the pulmonary artery is the first procedure performed because the infant's heart condition is poor. Prior to surgery, there are concerns that it may be difficult to switch the right pulmonary artery from the aorta to the main pulmonary artery, but this operation is safely performed through a median sternotomy. After that, it is relatively easy to move the left main bronchus from the esophagus to the stump of the esophagus fistula.

Seguier-Lipszyc et al. [12] reported a patient diagnosed after TEF surgery and was immediately reoperated.

Takamizawa et al. performed an operation to protect the left lung [25]. In the current case, both of the tracheobronchial anastomosis for CBPFM and the slide tracheoplasty for LCTS were successfully performed. This is the first report of a successful tracheobronchial reconstruction for a patient with an LCTS and CBPFM preserving the ipsilateral lung function.

## 12.8 Outcome

Yang et al. reported 8 patients died in 55 cases who underwent surgeries [7]. Unilateral pneumonectomy was performed in 6 patients in Group I, 11 patients in Group II, and 1 patient in Group IV. Three cases of group IA and four cases of group II received esophageal bronchial retransplantation. Twenty-four patients from Group IB, Group III, or Group IV had a lung resection or abnormal lung tissue and bronchial resection.

Four each were Group I, two were Group IB, and one was Group II and Group III. However, because the results of 15 cases (24.6%) were unknown, the mortality rate of 45 cases for which results were reported was 17.4%. Among survivors, 44.3% were reported as follow-up success. Eight cases (13.1%) had respiratory illnesses such as airway stenosis, tracheal softening, recurrent respiratory infections, and difficulty withdrawing from the ventilator. Post-pulmonary resection syndrome occurred in one case. In these series, seven patients underwent bronchial reconstruction. The longest follow-up period was 7 years. Two cases died (one during surgery and one 5 days after surgery). Three patients underwent multiple surgeries because of bronchial esophageal fissure, bronchial stenosis, difficulty eating, and tracheal stenosis with bronchial softening. Other complications included severe gastroesophageal reflux, anastomotic stenosis, and recurrent respiratory infections. Only two cases were reported to have no symptoms with normal growth on long-term follow-up.

## 12.9 Conclusion

For the treatment of this type of complex foregut anomaly, arriving at a correct diagnosis is the most important factor in determining the appropriate operative management. There are able to sort out the anatomy by radiologic imaging and bronchoscopy. Consequently, there are able to perform serial operations to successfully preserve the affected lung, air way and reconstruct the esophagus.

## References

1. Rokitansky C. Lehrbuch der pathologischen Anatomie. 3rd ed. Vienna; 1861. p. 44.
2. Rektorzik E. Ueber accessorische Lungenlapen. Wochenbl Z Ges Aerzte. 1861;17:4–6.
3. Pryce DM. Lower accessory pulmonary artery with intralobar sequestration of lung: a report of seven cases. J Pathol. 1946;58:457–67.
4. Weinbaum PJ, Bors-Koefoed R, Green K. Antenatal ultrasonographic findings in a case of intra-abdominal pulmonary sequestration. Obstet Gynecol. 1989;73:860–1.
5. Samuel M, Burge DM. Extra-lobar intra-abdominal pulmonary sequestration. Eur J Pediatr Surg. 1996;6:107–9.
6. Gerle RD, Jaretzki A 3rd, Ashley CA. Congenital bronchopulmonary foregut malformation. N Engl J Med. 1968;278:1413–9.
7. Yang G, Chen L, Xu C, Yuan M, Li Y. Congenital bronchopulmonary foregut malformation: systematic review of the literature. BMC Pediatr. 2019;19:305–12.

8. Srikanth MS, Ford EG, Stanley P, Mahour GH. Communicating bronchopulmonary foregut malformations: classification and embryogenesis. J Pediatr Surg. 1992;27:732–6.
9. Chiba T, Ohi R, Hayashi Y, et al. Bronchopulmonary foregut malformation in 3 infants-with special references to cases in childhood. Z Kinderchir. 1989;44:105–8.
10. Usui N, Kamata S, Ishikawa S, et al. Bronchial reconstruction for bronchopulmonary foregut malformation: a case report. J Pediatr Surg. 1995;30:1496–7.
11. Tsugawa J, Tsugawa C, Satoh S, et al. Communicating bronchopulmonary foregut malformation: particular emphasis on concomitant congenital tracheobronchial stenosis. Pediatr Surg Int. 2005;21:932–5.
12. Seguier-Lipszyc E, Dauger S, Malbezin S, et al. Reimplantation of oesophageal bronchus following a type III oesophageal atresia repair. Pediatr Surg Int. 2005;21:649–51.
13. Ryan DP, Muehrcke DD, Doopy DP, et al. Laryngotracheoesophageal cleft (type IV): management and repair of lesions beyond the carina. J Pediatr Surg. 1991;26:962–70.
14. Kawaguchi AL, Donahoe PK, Ryan DP, et al. Management and long- term follow-up of patients with types III and IV laryngotracheoesophageal clefts. J Pediatr Surg. 2005;40:158–65.
15. Saydam TC, Mychaliska GB, Harrison MR. Esophageal lung with multiple congenital anomalies: conundrums in diagnosis and management. J Pediatr Surg. 1999;34:615–8.
16. Lallemand D, Quignodon JF, Courtel JV. The anomalous origin of bronchus from the esophagus: report of three cases. Pediatr Radiol. 1996;26(3):179–82.
17. Michel JL, Revillon Y, Salakos C, et al. Successful bronchotracheal reconstruction in esophageal bronchus: two case reports. J Pediatr Surg. 1997;32:739–42.
18. Grosfeld JL, O'Neil JA, Fonkalsrud EW, et al. Pediatric surgery. 6th ed. Philadelphia: Mosby/Elsevier; 2006. p. 995–6.
19. Merei JM, Hutson JM. Embryogenesis of tracheo-esophageal anomalies: a review. Pediatr Surg Int. 2002;18:319–26.
20. Black MD, Bass J, Martin DJ, Carpenter BF. Intraabdominal pulmonary sequestration. J Pediatr Surg. 1983;26:1381–3.
21. Stallworth J, Campbell B, Carpenter C, et al. Communicating bronchopulmonary foregut malformation: a case report. J S C Med Assoc. 2004;100:278–80.
22. Morad NA, Al-Malki T, E-Tahir M. Intra-abdominal pulmonary sequestration: diagnostic difficulties. Pathology. 1997;29:218–20.
23. Garcia-Pena P, Lucaya J, Hendry GM, McAndrew PT, Duran C. Spontaneous involution of pulmonary sequestration in children: a report of two cases and review of the literature. Pediatr Radiol. 1998;28:266–70.
24. Shen KR, Wain JC, Wright CD, et al. Postpneumonectomy syndrome: surgical management and long-term results. J Thorac Cardiovasc Surg. 2008;135:1210–9.
25. Takamizawa S, Yoshizawa K, Machida M, et al. Successful tracheobronchial reconstruction of communicating bronchopulmonary foregut malformation and long segment congenital tracheal stenosis: a case report. J Pediatr Surg. 2012;47(9):E41–6.

# 13 Endoscopic Surgery for Pediatric Congenital Cystic Lung Disease

Hiroyuki Koga and Atsuyuki Yamataka

**Abstract**

Thoracoscopic pulmonary lobectomy is the treatment of choice for congenital pulmonary airway malformation and intralobar pulmonary sequestration in infants and children, both of which are now commonly diagnosed prenatally. The timing of surgery is somewhat controversial in asymptomatic cases with small isolated lesions. Thorough understanding of anatomic relations preoperatively is vital for successful outcome and thin-slice computed tomography with three-dimensional reconstruction of vessels is valuable. Judicious placement of trocars and switching instruments between trocars improves visualization and safety. Incomplete fissures and history of chest infections are most problematic.

**Keywords**

Thoracoscopic surgery · Pulmonary lobectomy · Congenital cystic lung disease · Congenital pulmonary airway malformation · Sequestration

H. Koga · A. Yamataka (✉)
Department of Pediatric General and Urogenital Surgery, Juntendo University School of Medicine, Tokyo, Japan
e-mail: h-koga@juntendo.ac.jp; yama@juntendo.ac.jp

## 13.1 Introduction

Our aim is to present the specific techniques for commonly performed thoracoscopic pulmonary lobectomy (TPL) rather than discuss technical options for pulmonary resection in infants and children as can be found in major surgery textbooks [1, 2]. We will describe our TPL techniques in infants and children in detail, including relevant tips and advice and use diagrams/figures where possible to improve understanding and enhance practical application.

## 13.2 Indications for Surgery

Currently, TPL is the treatment of choice for congenital cystic lung diseases, such as congenital pulmonary airway malformation (CPAM) and intralobar pulmonary sequestration (ILPS) [3].

## 13.3 Preoperative Imaging Studies

### 13.3.1 Computerized Tomography

In prenatally diagnosed cases of CPAM/ILPS, computerized tomography (CT) with or without contrast is performed as early after delivery as is practical to confirm the diagnosis. Thin-slice contrast CT is particularly valuable for assessing



H. Sago et al. (eds.), *Congenital Cystic Lung Disease*, https://doi.org/10.1007/978-981-15-5175-8_13

the anatomic relations of a lesion/lesions in relation to the pulmonary arteries and veins, the bronchi, as well as confirming the status of fissures between the upper and lower lobes of the left lung, and between the upper and lower (Fig. 13.1), upper and middle, and middle and lower lobes of the right lung. Fissure appearance may not always be accurate on CT, with an incomplete fissure appearing complete, so surgeons must be constantly aware that an incomplete fissure may be present at surgery. The anatomy of the pulmonary arteries must be understood, and any variations or anomalies must be delineated preoperatively. This is most important in the left upper lobe, because variations are common; for example, mediastinal A4 and A5 should be identified accurately on preoperative CT, and if they are located behind A3, they could be injured inadvertently during left upper lobe TPL. Mediastinal A4 and A5 are present in 30% of cases (Fig. 13.2); purely mediastinal in 18% and mediastinal and otherwise in 12% [4]. In ILPS cases, blood flow from a feeding artery to a draining vein can be reconstructed three dimensionally from thin-slice contrast CT images and provide valuable insight into the hemodynamics of a sequestration. It is known that 73% of feeding arteries originate from the abdominal aorta, and multiple feeding arteries are found in 15% of sequestrations [2]. The recommended timing for the final preoperative thin-slice contrast CT should be less than 1 month prior to TPL.

### 13.3.2 Chest X-Ray Radiography

Chest X-ray radiography (CXR) is also taken after delivery as a reference for comparison of cyst size during subsequent follow-up. TPL is indicated if CXR shows no change in the size of

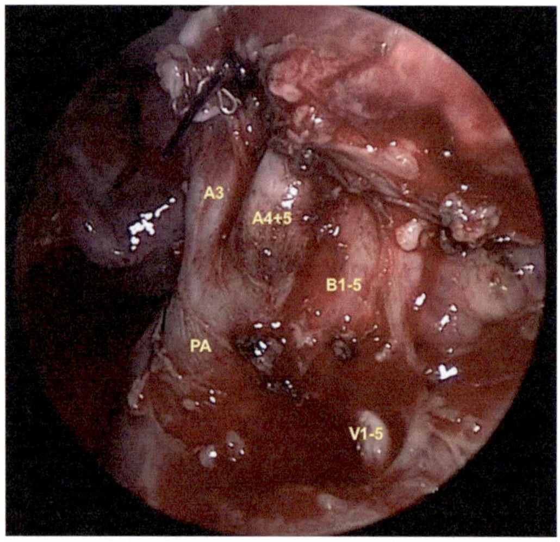


**Fig. 13.2** Mediastinal A4+5 behind A3 during a left upper lobectomy. PA, B1-5, and V1-5 represent pulmonary artery, upper lobe bronchus, and superior pulmonary vein (already divided by stapling), respectively

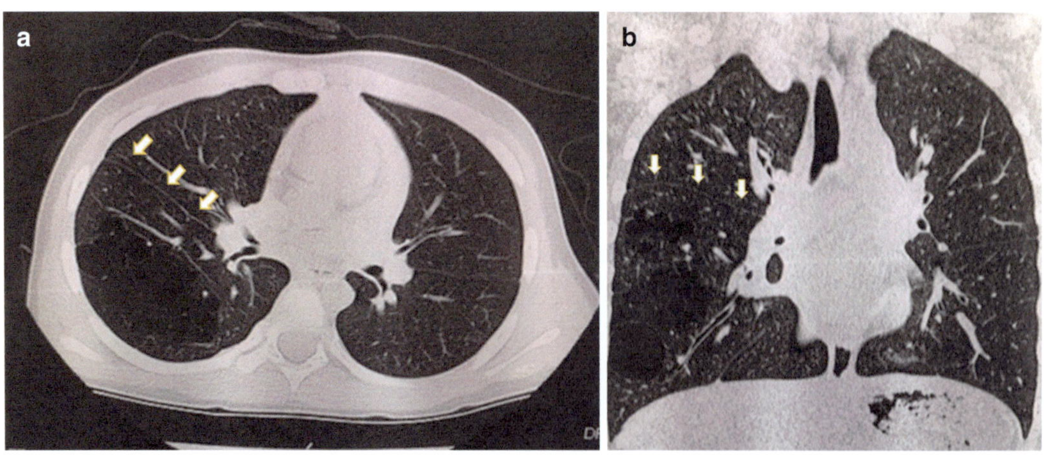


**Fig. 13.1** A complete fissure (arrowheads) between the left upper and lower lobes shown on computer tomography (**a**: axial view; **b**: sagittal view)

a large lesion or increase in the size of a large lesion. If a lesion is small to moderate on CXR, the timing of TPL is controversial.

## 13.4 Factors that Will Affect Surgery

### 13.4.1 Status of Fissures

The greatest obstacle to successful TPL is the status of the fissures between lung lobes. Fissures may be complete, incomplete, or absent (Fig. 13.3), and the extent of abnormal can vary. If a fissure is complete, lobes are separated only by pleura and all anatomic structures in the fissure are readily visible (Fig. 13.4), facilitating TPL. If a fissure is incomplete, TPL is most challenging, because anatomic relations can vary greatly and successful TPL requires thorough knowledge of as many variations as possible. If a fissure is completely absent, there is only an expanse of lung parenchyma visible. A detailed description of TPL when a fissure is absent will be presented for each lobe later, but the general concept is that the pulmonary veins and bronchi to the affected lobe and mediastinal pulmonary artery branches are divided first, followed by the branches of the lobar pulmonary artery to the affected lobe, and finally, the fused parenchyma constituting the absent fissure between the two lobes is divided with a stapler [5, 6].

### 13.4.2 Past History of Chest Infections

From experience, and research comparing blood loss during surgery and intra-/postoperative complication rates of TPL in relation to a past history of chest infections [7], TPL is easier to perform in the absence of a past history of chest infections although there were no significant differences in intraoperative blood loss or incidence of complications.

### 13.4.3 Other Factors

The most relevant other factors are also anatomic. Variation in pulmonary arteries, such as the presence of mediastinal A4 and A5 in the left upper lobe as mentioned earlier (Fig. 13.2), and the level at which A6 and B6 branch to the superior

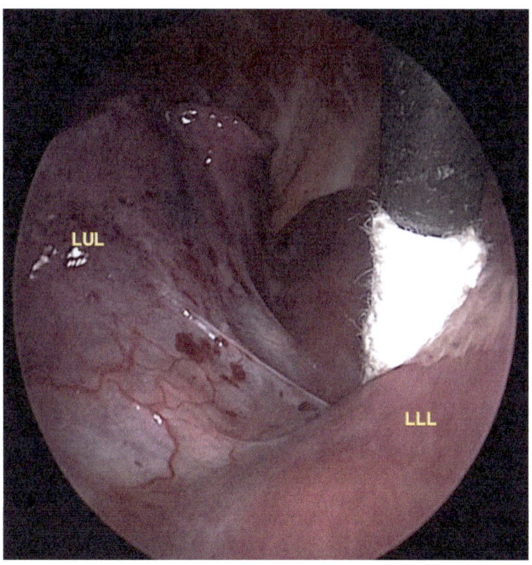


**Fig. 13.3** Intraoperative photo showing an absent fissure between the left upper (LUL) and left lower (LLL) lobes. Thus the lobar pulmonary artery between LUL and LLL cannot be identified at all

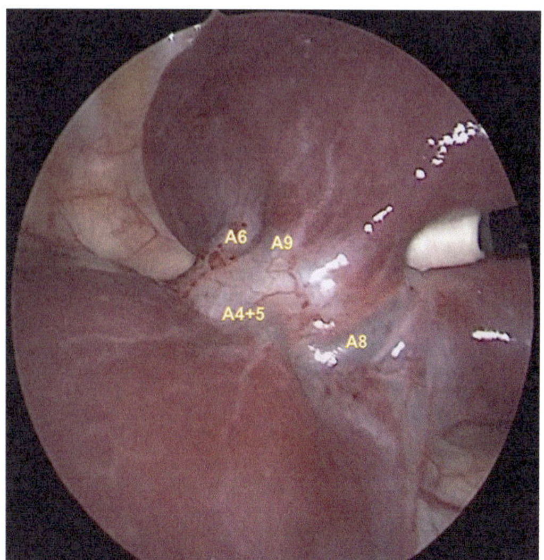


**Fig. 13.4** Intraoperative photo showing a lobar pulmonary artery (asterisk), A4+5, and A8, visible in a complete fissure

segment of the right lower lobe will affect operative time and must be confirmed/excluded preoperatively. There is no way to do this intraoperatively and poor understanding of the anatomy of a cystic lesion may have dire consequences. Before TPL, surgeons should know exactly how many feeding arteries to an ILPS originate from the aorta and know their respective lengths to ensure that an ILPS is treated thoroughly. There seem to be an abundance of lymph nodes in infants and children with CPAM or ILPS, even in the absence of a past history of chest infections, which is probably a consequence of chronic asymptomatic inflammation in the affected lobe. Lymph nodes can be an annoying source of minor bleeding which during TPL is nothing but detrimental, because the operative field is compromised. The ideal TPL should be bloodless. Lymph nodes should be cauterized while being dissected.

## 13.5 Tips for Facilitating TPL

### 13.5.1 Patient Preparation and Positioning

After anesthetization, the patient is placed in the lateral position, prepped, and draped. The patient should be placed toward the edge of the operating table in front of the operating surgeon to enhance maneuverability and prevent instruments from hitting the table. Operative devices, such as electrocautery and LigaSure™ (Covidien, Mansfield, MA, USA), should not be placed between the patient or the surgeon to keep the area between the patient and surgeon as open as possible. If there is not enough space, handheld instruments may hit operative devices.

### 13.5.2 Trocar Insertion

An optical trocar is used as the initial trocar and is placed slightly posterior to the posterior axillary line using a closed technique 1 cm below the inferior angle of the scapula. The closed technique allows artificial pneumothorax to be maintained nicely, because there is no leakage of $CO_2$ from around the trocar at the trocar site, thus facilitating complete collapse of the lung throughout the entire TPL procedure. Pneumothorax is maintained with $CO_2$ at an insufflation pressure of 4–6 mmHg and flow rate of 0.5–1.5 L/min to collapse the ipsilateral lung.

### 13.5.3 Trocar Positions and Switching Instruments

Trocar positions for a left lower lobectomy are shown in Fig. 13.5. The initial trocar is used for lung retraction. Trocars for a 5 mm 30° scope, the surgeon's left hand, and the surgeon's right hand are placed in the sixth, fourth, and eighth intercostal spaces in the anterior axillary line, respectively (Fig. 13.5c, d). Most surgeons perform a lower lobe lobectomy by placing the scope in the sixth intercostal space (Fig. 13.5c) for the entire procedure which is suitable for dissecting the interlobar pulmonary artery (Fig. 13.5a) but limits visualization because by placing the scope in the sixth intercostal space, dissection progresses from anterior to posterior, which prevents the posterior aspects of the bronchi and pulmonary veins, as well as the posterior mediastinum from being viewed readily and could be unsafe. An extra trocar (asterisk in Fig. 13.5) placed in the tenth intercostal space in the posterior axillary line during dissection or inspection of vital structures, such as the pulmonary veins, bronchus, and feeding artery/arteries gives a posterior perspective as well as enabling the pulmonary artery, aortic arch, and the vagus nerve to be observed in their entirety, ensuring the safety and reliability of TPL. Thus, during dissection of a feeding artery (Fig. 13.5b) originating from the aorta and dissection of the posterior wall of the inferior pulmonary vein and left bronchus we switch the scope from the eighth intercostal space trocar to the sixth intercostal space trocar (Fig. 13.5d), and the left-hand instrument from the sixth intercostal space trocar to the fourth intercostal space trocar, as required. Switching instruments also contributes to minimizing blood loss during TPL.

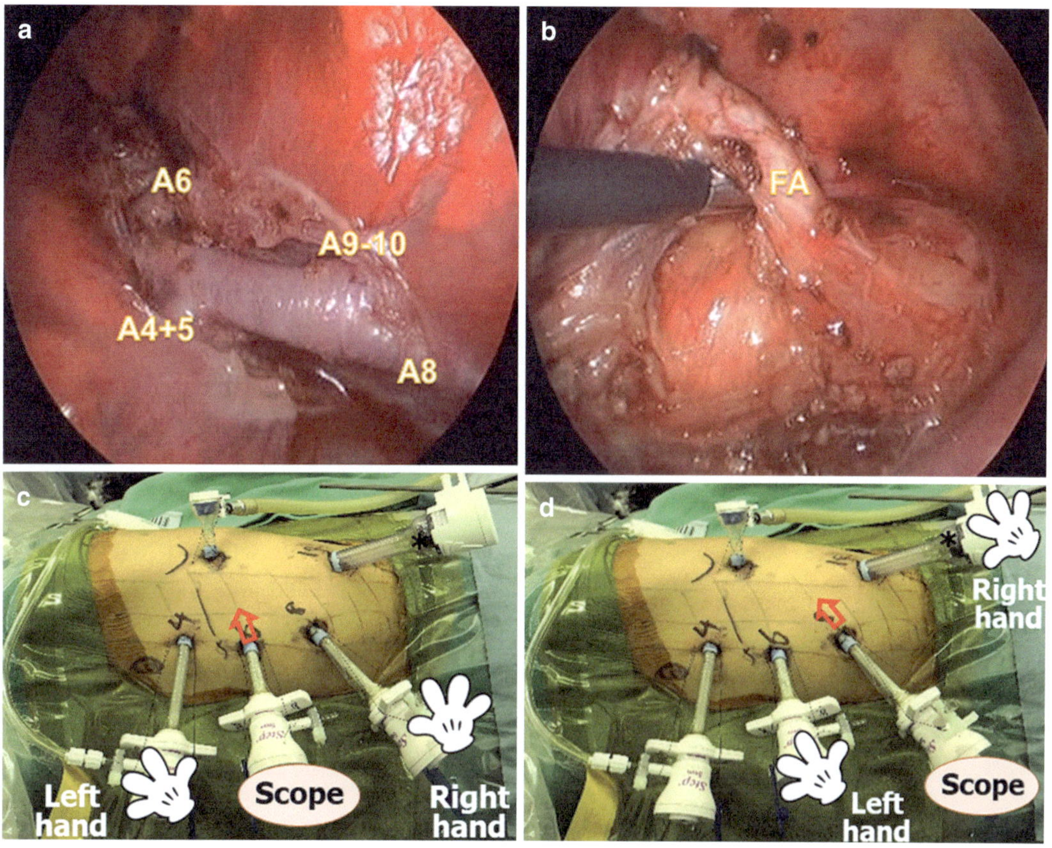


**Fig. 13.5** Trocar positions for a left lower lobectomy. Note the extra trocar (asterisk) in the tenth intercostal space. This extra trocar facilitates safe dissection of a feeding artery (FA) originating from the aorta (**b**) and the posterior aspects of the inferior pulmonary vein and left bronchus (**d**). It is also valuable for observing the pulmonary artery aortic arch and course of the vagus nerve. Most surgeons perform a lower lobe lobectomy by placing the scope in the sixth intercostal space (**c**) for the entire procedure without using an extra trocar. While this is suitable for dissecting A8-10 (**a**), placing an extra trocar in the tenth intercostal space to prevent dissection from progressing from anterior to posterior without viewing the posterior mediastinum readily, is safer and highly recommended

Specifically, for an upper lobectomy on either side, trocar positions are one intercostal space higher than for a lower lobectomy, i.e., third, fifth, seventh, and ninth intercostal spaces (Fig. 13.6). When the scope is switched from the fifth intercostal space trocar (Fig. 13.6a) to a trocar in either the seventh or ninth intercostal spaces (Fig. 13.6b, c), A1+2, A3, and A6 which is the only segmental pulmonary artery located posterolateral to the lobar pulmonary artery can be seen readily (Fig. 13.7), ensuring safer TPL. Without an extra trocar placed in the ninth intercostal space, the pulmonary hilum cannot be viewed posteriorly at all, with the result that the entire TPL will be performed only in the anterior–posterior plane (Fig. 13.6a) which is not ideal, especially if a fissure is incomplete.

For a middle lobectomy, the trocars for the right hand, the scope, and the left hand are placed in the fourth, fifth, and seventh intercostal spaces in the right anterior axillary line, respectively. To create more space between the scope trocar and the right-hand trocar, the scope trocar can be placed slightly more anteriorly than the right-hand trocar which will prevent the scope and the right-hand instrument from hitting each other.

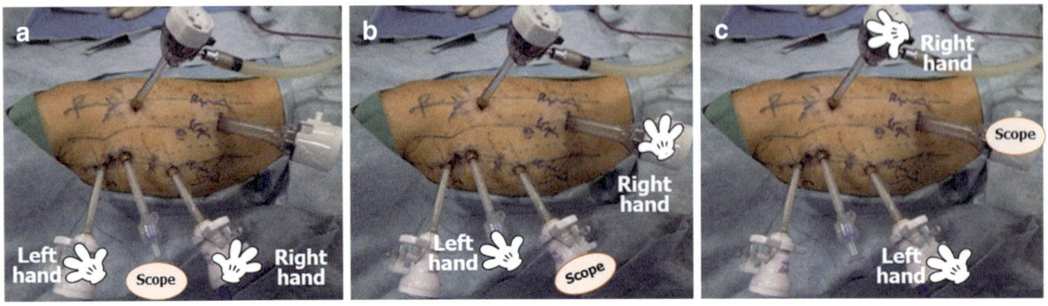


**Fig. 13.6** For an upper lobectomy, all trocar positions are one intercostal space higher, i.e., the third, fifth, seventh, and ninth intercostal spaces. The scope is switched from the fifth intercostal space trocar (**a**) to a trocar in either the seventh or ninth intercostal spaces (**b**, **c**), to view the entire course of the lobar pulmonary artery as well as the pulmonary hilum from the posterior mediastinum

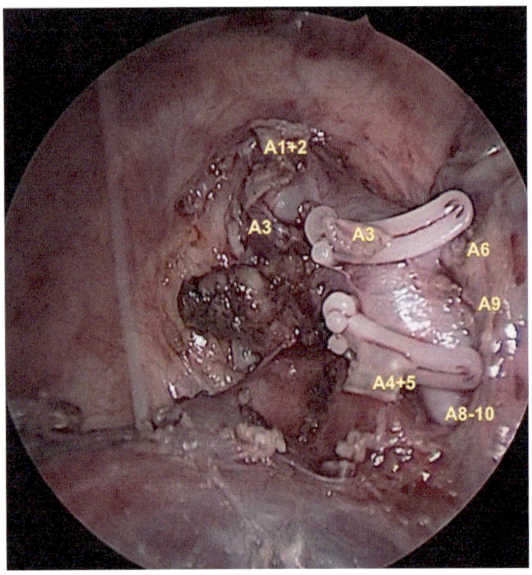


**Fig. 13.7** When the scope is switched from the trocar in the fifth intercostal space to either one of the trocars in the seventh or ninth intercostal space, A1+2 and A3 can be observed more easily enhancing the safety of TPL

## 13.6 Treating an Incomplete Fissure

In general, during TPL in infants and children, the view through the scope is from front to back and limited by the small size of the thorax, which means treating an incomplete fissure located anteriorly, such as an incomplete fissure between S4+5 and S8 in the left lung, or between the upper and middle lobes in the right lung, or between the middle and lower lobes in the right lung, is more difficult than treating an incomplete fissure located posteriorly, such as an incomplete fissure between S1+2 and S6 in the left lung, or between the upper and lower lobes in the right lung.

### 13.6.1 Right Lung

The interlobar pulmonary artery at the confluence of the oblique and horizontal fissures can usually be exposed without difficulty even if a fissure is incomplete, because the parenchyma overlying it is usually thin. Once A8, A9, and A10 have been identified, the pleura and thin parenchyma over A8 can be incised using electrocautery or LigaSure™ allowing A6, A7, ascending A2, A4, and A5 to be displayed. To divide an incomplete fissure between the right upper and lower lobes, the interlobar pulmonary artery must be exposed (Fig. 13.8a) and a tunnel toward the posterior mediastinum created by dissecting the right pulmonary artery along with its wall beneath the pulmonary artery sheath, taking great care not to injure A6 and ascending A2 (Fig. 13.8b). The lung parenchyma in the incomplete fissure is then divided using an Enseal® device (Ethicon Endo-Surgery, Inc., Cincinnati, OH, USA) (Fig. 13.8c) rather than a LigaSure™ device [8] because with Enseal®, sealing occurs slowly while apposing the tips of the device, thus

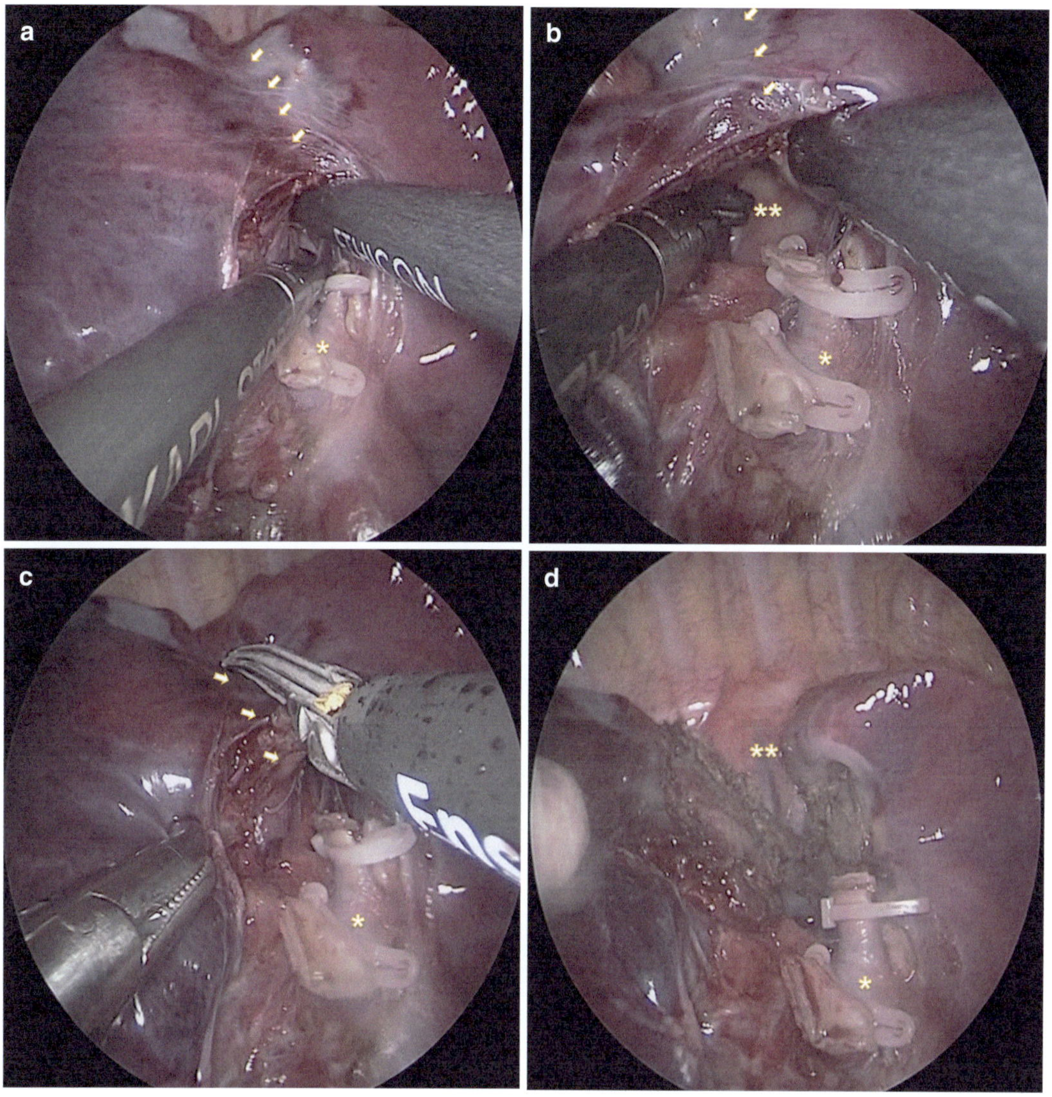

**Fig. 13.8** A tunnel being created between a lobar pulmonary artery and the lung parenchyma in an incomplete fissure moving toward the posterior mediastinum (**a**). The tunnel reaching the posterior mediastinum (**b**). Enseal® has been applied to divide thick lung parenchyma in an incomplete fissure (**c**). The incomplete fissure has been treated without any bleeding or air leakage (**d**). The asterisk indicates a lobar pulmonary artery. Double asterisks indicate the posterior mediastinum. Arrows indicate thick lung parenchyma in an incomplete fissure

minimizing bleeding, crushing, tearing, and air leakage, while with LigaSure™, sealing starts after the tips of the device are apposed and there can be some tissue damage prior to sealing particularly if tissue is thick, as the lung parenchyma in an incomplete fissure is apt to be. From experience, there is less bleeding and less air leakage with Enseal® during TPL and the resulting seal seems stronger than with LigaSure™ [8]. Irrespective of the device used, the seal of the divided edge must be checked thoroughly for completeness, hemostasis, and air leakage (Fig. 13.8d).

For dividing lung parenchyma in an incomplete fissure between the middle and lower lobes or between the upper and middle lobes, a tunnel is created below the lung parenchyma between the middle and lower lobes or below the lung parenchyma between the upper and middle lobes, respectively, by dissecting carefully between the pulmonary hilum in the anterior mediastinum and the site of the interlobar pulmonary artery, with supplementary circumferential dissection of bronchi as required.

### 13.6.2 Left Lung

The left lung is treated similarly to the right lung. At the mid-portion of the oblique fissure, lobar pulmonary arteries can usually be exposed without difficulty even in the presence of an incomplete fissure. Once the lobar pulmonary arteries have been exposed, A8-10, A5, and A4 are identified anteriorly, and A6 and A1+2 are identified posteriorly. An incomplete fissure between S1+2 and S6 can be divided by creating a tunnel by dissecting underneath the lobar pulmonary artery sheath toward the posterior mediastinum, taking great care not to injure A1+2 and A6. Incising the pleura over the posterior aspect of the pulmonary hilum is helpful for creating the tunnel, and is made possible by switching the scope from the fifth intercostal space to the seventh or ninth intercostal spaces (Fig. 13.6b, c). For division of an incomplete fissure between S4+5 and S8, a tunnel is created carefully from the pulmonary hilum between the superior and inferior pulmonary veins in the anterior mediastinum to superior to the origin of A8. The bronchus can be identified between the superior and inferior pulmonary veins by observing from the ventral aspect of the pulmonary hilum. A8 may be identified by burrowing along the bronchus toward the external aspect of the lung. Once the tunnel is created, the lung parenchyma of the incomplete fissure may be divided using Enseal®.

### 13.6.3 Delivering the Excised Lung

The posterolateral side trocar site slightly below the inferior angle of the scapula is enlarged to 1.5 cm. This wound is on the posterolateral side of the patient and is not visible when the patient is viewed anteriorly.

### 13.6.4 Stapling the Bronchus

The smallest sized stapler currently available in Japan is 5 mm with white cartridges with 1 mm staples, fired in two rows. Gray cartridges with 0.75 mm staples are available for 10 mm staplers but not for 5 mm staplers. While a 5 mm stapler is attractive because of its smaller size, 1 mm staples could cause bleeding in thin tissues. For stapling a bronchus, an Endopath® Endocutter ETS (Ethicon Endo-Surgery, Inc., Cincinnati OH) or Endo GIA™ Curved Tip Reload with Tri-Staple™ Technology (Medtronic plc., Dublin, Ireland) is applied to the bronchus of the affected lobe and the lung is inflated to check for any compromise to aeration of the rest of the bronchial tree before firing the stapler. If the stapler is obstructing some other part of the bronchial tree, the stapler should be reapplied or the bronchus of the affected lung should be clipped with Hem-o-lok (Teleflex Medical, NC, USA) or stapled, separately, i.e., during left lower lobectomy, the bronchus to the superior segment must be stapled before the bronchus to the basal segments to prevent compromise of airflow to the rest of the lung (Fig. 13.9).

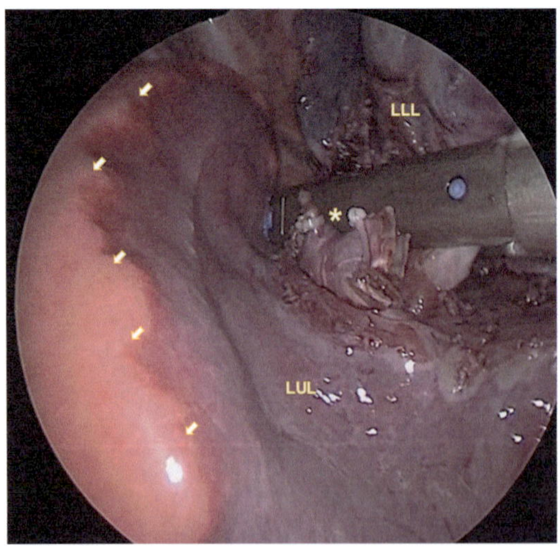


**Fig. 13.9** Stapling of bronchi during a left lower lobectomy. The left upper lobe should be ventilated before firing the stapler (asterisk) on the affected left lower lobe (LLL) to ensure that there is no compromise to aeration (arrows) of the remaining left upper lobe (LUL)

## 13.7 Surgical Techniques for TPL

### 13.7.1 Left Lower Lobectomy

Check the fissure is between the lingula and S8 and between S1+2 and S6 for completeness. Usually, if the latter fissure is incomplete, the fissure is probably going to be absent. Identify the lobar pulmonary artery (Fig. 13.4). In ILPS cases, identify the feeding artery/arteries. The anatomy of the feeding artery/arteries should be studied thoroughly using three-dimensional images reconstructed from preoperative thin slice contrast CT to confirm their length, thickness, and origin; over 70% of feeding arteries originate from the abdominal aorta and may be multiple in 15% of cases [2]. The pleura over the lobar pulmonary artery is incised, and the sheath of the artery is incised carefully with a right-angled tip electrocautery device, Endopath® Probe Plus II (Ethicon Endo-Surgery, LLC) which is extremely useful for this purpose, because it has a switch on the handle for both cutting and coagulation as well as suction and irrigation functions. Identify A4+5 and A8 anteriorly and A6 which arises posterolateral to the lobar pulmonary artery. Be aware that A4+5 in the upper lobe lingula may originate from A8 in the lower lobe, and A1+2 in the upper lobe may originate from A6 in the lower lobe. If the fissure between S1+2 and S6 is incomplete, a space between the lobar pulmonary artery and the fused lung parenchyma of the incomplete fissure is dissected free by creating a tunnel to the posterior mediastinum, taking great care not to injure A6 and A1+2. If the fissure between S4+5 and S8 is incomplete, a tunnel between the lobar pulmonary artery and the fused lung parenchyma is created from the pulmonary hilum in the anterior mediastinum to where the lobar pulmonary artery was mobilized. Fused lung parenchyma is divided using Enseal®. A8-10 are usually divided during the process of tunneling which facilitates further tunneling. A6 to the superior segment of the lower lobe is usually divided after the lung parenchyma comprising an incomplete fissure has been divided. A8-10 and A6 are clipped proximally with an endoscopic clip, such as Hem-o-lok, Endo Clip™ III 5 mm Clip Applier (Medtronic, plc., Dublin, Ireland), sealed with LigaSure™ distally and divided. A6 is clipped separately from A8-10 and divided. The basilar segmental artery can usually be clipped and divided en bloc. After dividing the inferior pulmonary ligament with electrocautery superiorly to the level of the inferior pulmonary vein, the inferior pulmonary vein is mobilized, and the pleura is divided along the pericardial reflection. The inferior pulmonary veins are clipped proximally and divided distally with LigaSure®, or divided with a stapler, along their most medial aspect to decrease potential dead space for left atrial clot formation. A stapler or Hem-o-lok clip is then applied to the bronchial tree of the lower lobe; however, if the B6 bifurcation is considerably proximal, B6 and B8-10 should be stapled or clipped separately to prevent stenosis of the bronchus to the upper lobe. If the bronchi of the superior and basal segments are stapled together, the bronchus of the upper lobe may be compromised. The anesthetist is asked to inflate the upper lobe to check that there is no compromise to aeration. Bronchial arteries run posterior to the bronchial tree, so observing the posterior aspect of the left lower lobe bronchus through a trocar in the eighth or tenth intercostal space is extremely useful when it is time to treat the bronchial arteries (Fig. 13.6b, c).

### 13.7.2 Right Lower Lobectomy

Begin dissection at the confluence of fissures and identify the interlobar pulmonary artery or a branch of it (usually A8). Although this artery lies deep in the region of the confluence of the oblique and horizontal fissures, exposure is usually possible by retracting the upper lobe superiorly and the lower lobe inferiorly using forceps inserted through the trocar below the scapula and the trocar in the ninth or tenth intercostal spaces. Incise the visceral pleura over the interlobar pulmonary artery or its branches and mobilize the interlobar pulmonary artery. Take note of the location of the superior segmental branch of A6, as A6 generally lies directly opposite middle lobe branches A4 and A5; however, it might bifurcate proximal to the middle lobe branches. A6 must be clipped separately and divided after which the basilar segmental arteries (A7-10) are usually clipped and divided en bloc. Segmental pulmonary artery branches are divided in the same way as described in the section on left lower lobectomy. Keep in mind that A4 to the middle lobe may originate from A8.

Next, mobilize and divide the pulmonary ligament and divide the pleural reflection along the inferior half of the hilum to expose the inferior pulmonary vein and bronchus intermedius. After mobilizing the inferior pulmonary vein, clip or staple it at the peritoneal reflection. Be aware that V6 may drain anomalously into the left atrium independently from other basilar vein branches (B7-10) in which case V2 may drain anomalously into the anomalous V6. Finally, after identifying and mobilizing the bronchus to the lower lobe, divide it with a stapler or clip, checking before firing to ascertain that stapling will not compromise aeration of the middle lobe. It may be necessary to protect the middle lobe by clipping/stapling the bronchus (B6) to the superior segment of the lower lobe separately from basilar segment bronchi (B7-10), especially if the B6 bifurcation is proximal to the middle lobe bronchi B4 and B5. Remember that A6 to the superior segment of the lower lobe bifurcates proximal to A4 and A5 to the middle lobe and B6 almost always will bifurcates proximal to the middle lobe bronchus.

If a fissure is incomplete, divide the lung parenchyma in the fissure using Enseal® or an endoscopic stapler. While creating a tunnel from the area of arterial dissection at the confluence of the oblique and horizontal fissures to the posterior mediastinum for applying Enseal® or a stapler to separate the incomplete fissure, A6 and ascending A2 must be identified with care to prevent injuring these two vessels. Be aware that ascending A2 may originate from A6.

### 13.7.3 Left Upper Lobectomy

This is probably the most difficult lobectomy [9]. Identify mediastinal A3 and the superior pulmonary vein at the pulmonary hilum (Fig. 13.10a). Start dissecting the pulmonary artery proximally to divide the interlobar A1+2 and A3 arteries. Remember interlobar A1+2 may originate from

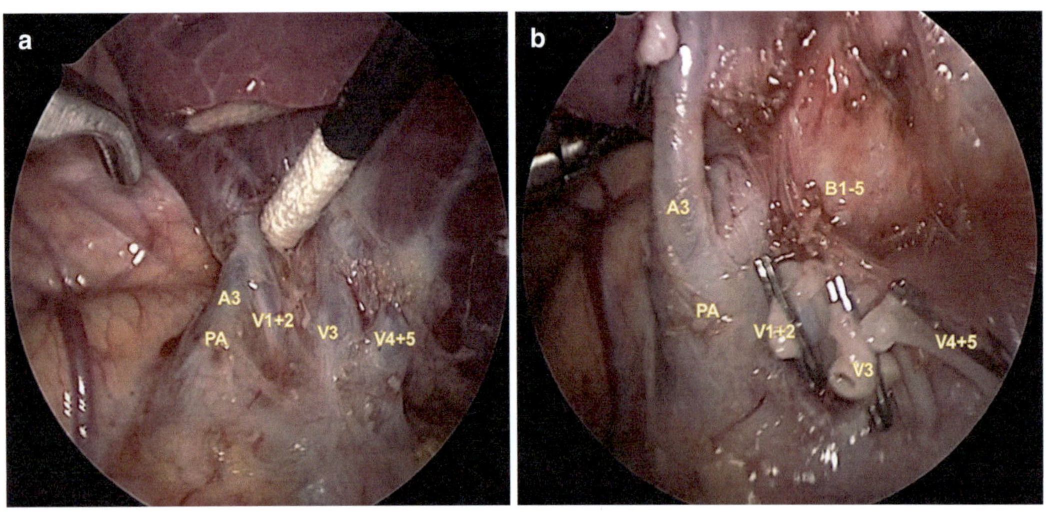


**Fig. 13.10** Mediastinal A3 is short pedicled and lies behind superior pulmonary vein branches V1+2 initially (**a**). After exposing A3 from the lung parenchyma, the pedicle was longer (**b**). Mediastinal pulmonary artery (PA) branch A3 after division of superior pulmonary veins branches V1+2, V3, and V4+5 ready to be clipped, sealed, and divided. B1-5 indicates the superior lobe bronchus

A6 to the lower lobe. Mobilize mediastinal A3 and dissect it free, taking great care not to injure it as it originates proximally from the pulmonary artery and is short pedicled. Bleeding from A3 can be fatal. Because of this, we strongly recommend dividing mediastinal V1+2 and V3 of the superior pulmonary vein first and then dissecting the anterior aspect of the upper lobe bronchus to expose mediastinal A3 fully (Fig. 13.10b). Then, it can be clipped, sealed, and divided. After division of mediastinal A3, A1+2, and V1–V3, attention is paid to segmental branches in the oblique fissure. If the posterior aspect of the oblique fissure is incomplete, Enseal® is used to complete the fissure. Identify A4+ 5 and A8-10 anteriorly and A6 posteriorly. For this purpose, the scope should be switched at some stage, from the trocar in the fifth intercostal space to a trocar in either the seventh or ninth intercostal spaces to allow the entire lobar pulmonary artery to be viewed and ensure safe division of A1+2 and A3 (Fig. 13.6). Be aware that mediastinal A4 or A5 are present in 30% of cases [4] and may be present behind the superior pulmonary vein, caudal to A3 (Fig. 13.2). A5 in the upper lobe may originate from A8 in the lower lobe. Divide A4 and A5.

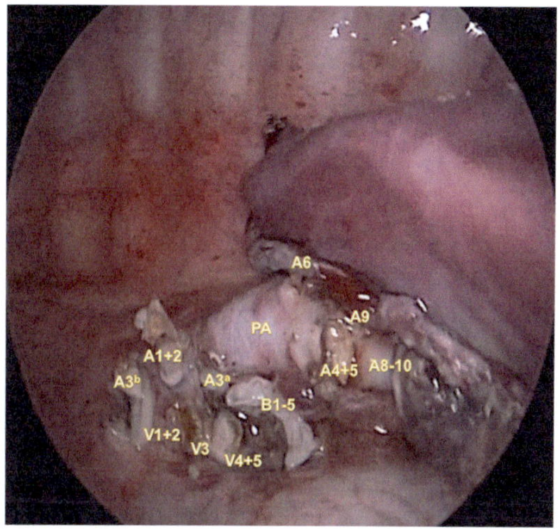


**Fig. 13.11** Anatomic relations at the pulmonary hilum after left upper lobectomy. Keep in mind that the posterior aspect of superior pulmonary veins V1-5 is closely attached to B1-5 bronchi to the left upper lobe. In cases with a past history of chest infections, there may be dense adhesions between the superior pulmonary vein and the bronchus and great care is required to prevent injury to the posterior aspect of the superior pulmonary vein during dissection. In addition, keep in mind that the pulmonary artery (PA) lies posterior to upper lobe bronchi B1-5. A1-10 are shown

During mobilization and dissection of V1+2 and V3, keep in mind that the posterior wall of the superior pulmonary vein is closely attached to the bronchus to the upper lobe (Fig. 13.11). In cases with a past history of chest infections, there may be dense adhesions between the superior pulmonary vein and the bronchus and great care is required not to injure the posterior wall of the superior pulmonary vein during dissection. Arteries and veins are clipped, sealed, and divided as mentioned earlier.

After division of V4 and V5 of the superior pulmonary vein, the bronchus to the upper lobe is mobilized, cleaned, and divided with a stapler or clip. Keep in mind that the posterior wall of the upper lobe bronchus is close to the pulmonary artery (Fig. 13.11), so dissecting the upper lobe bronchus with the scope in either the seventh or ninth intercostal spaces will improve safety, because the posterior aspect of the upper lobe bronchus and the entire pulmonary artery can be observed. The upper lobe bronchus is divided with a stapler or clip taking care to ensure that there is no compromise to aeration of the lower lobe.

### 13.7.4 Right Upper Lobectomy

While retracting the upper lobe inferiorly and posteriorly, divide the pleura around the pulmonary hilum in the anterior mediastinum. Identify the superior pulmonary vein and dissect along it distally to the lung parenchyma and mobilize it in the appropriate plane. Identify and preserve the middle lobe veins which typically enter the superior pulmonary vein. Be aware of aberrant venous drainage, including direct connections to the vena cava, that are often mentioned in textbooks, but which we have never seen personally. The presence of aberrant vessels should always be checked for, despite their rarity.

The pulmonary artery lies just posterior and superior to the superior pulmonary vein. Mobilize

A1-3 to the upper lobe. Successful mobilization of A1-3 requires care and concentration. Before commencing dissection, divide the apical segmental vein V1 that crosses A1-3 to improve exposure. Carefully dissect, clip, seal, and divide A1-3. Next, divide the remaining superior pulmonary vein branches, V2 and V3, separately by clipping proximally and sealing distally. V2 may lie deep between V1 and V3 and requires careful dissection. Once the superior pulmonary veins V1-3 are divided, the distal pulmonary artery and its branches can be visualized readily. Identify the remaining segmental branch, the posterior ascending branch (ascending A2, present in 90% of cases) which can be approached either from the anterior mediastinum in a retrograde fashion or from the oblique fissure between the upper and lower lobes, and the middle lobe branches, A4 and A5.

The course of the horizontal fissure (which is usually poorly defined) can be identified by making a tunnel from where V1-3 were divided to superior to A4+5. Use Enseal® to seal the lung parenchyma along the tunnel to complete the horizontal fissure. The technique for separating an incomplete fissure between lobes is also mentioned in the section "Treating an incomplete fissure."

The bronchus to the upper lobe is at an angle of almost 90° to the main stem bronchus and applying a clip or setting a stapler appropriately are easy. In the mediastinum, and at the hilum of a lung, bronchi are the most posterior of the major structures and small bronchial arteries and veins are associated intimately with them posteriorly. Prevention of bleeding from bronchial vessels is mandatory.

Care must be taken when dividing the pleural reflection to expose the bronchial tree, because the right vagus nerve associated with the esophagus lies just posterior to the line of pleural division.

### 13.7.5 Right Middle Lobe Lobectomy

Begin dissection at the confluence of the oblique and horizontal fissures where the interlobar pulmonary artery or its branches can be identified readily. There will be two branches to the middle lobe coming directly off the interlobar pulmonary artery. Keep in mind that A4 may originate from A7+8 to the basal segments of the lower lobe and that A3 may originate from A4+5.

Retract the middle lobe upward and posteriorly and divide the anterior mediastinal pleura posterior to the phrenic nerve to expose the superior pulmonary vein. Identify pulmonary vein branches V4 and V5, clip proximally with a Hem-o-lok clip, seal distally with LigaSure™, and divide. A stapler can be used in larger children, but not in infants with small thoracic cavities. Be aware that V4 or V4+5 may originate from the inferior pulmonary vein.

The oblique fissure is usually well developed and needs only minimal dissection to separate the middle lobe from the lower lobe. However, if the horizontal fissure is incomplete, a tunnel for passage of an Enseal® device or stapler from the anterior mediastinum, where V4 and V5 were divided, through to where A4 and A5 were dissected should be created to separate the middle lobe from the upper lobe. If the direction of this tunnel is superior after mobilizing B4+5, the tunnel will be between the upper and middle lobes, and if the direction of the tunnel is inferior after mobilizing B4+5, the tunnel will be between the middle and upper lobes.

Clean the bronchus and divide it with a clip in infants or a stapler in larger children. Before finalizing division of the bronchus with a clip or stapler, inflate the lung to ensure that the planned point of division will not interfere with aeration of the rest of the lung.

## 13.8 Postoperative Care

A chest tube is inserted one intercostal space above the lowest intercostal space used for trocar placement to ensure an air-tight seal around the chest tube and exteriorized through the lowest trocar wound. The tube is connected to 10 cm $H_2O$ suction and left in situ overnight. If there is no air leak after surgery, the chest tube is water-sealed the next morning, and a CXR is taken 6 h later. If the CXR is normal, the tube is clamped, and another CXR is taken the next morning. If the CXR is again normal, the tube is removed. A cephalosporin antibiotic is administered for 24 h postoperatively. Pain is usually controlled adequately by an intravenous narcotic for 24–36 h postoperatively. A thoracic epidural is rarely required. A regular diet is resumed on the day of surgery or from the morning after surgery. Patients are usually ready for discharge to home on day-3 after TPL when there is no air leakage.

## 13.9 The Authors' Experience

The authors have performed 55 TPL for CPAM/ILPS; 24 females and 31 male, between 2009 and 2018. Mean age and mean weight at TPL were 2.7 (0.1–8.5) years, and 12.3 (3.0–24.3) kg, respectively. Of these, 40 cases (72%) were diagnosed prenatally, and 14 cases (25%) had a history of preoperative infections. Types of TPL performed were: left upper lobe ($n = 8$), left lower lobe ($n = 18$), right upper lobe ($n = 1$), right upper lobe/right middle lobe ($n = 2$), right middle lobe/right lower lobe ($n = 1$), right middle lobe ($n = 5$), and right lower lobe ($n = 20$). Pulmonary fissures were absent or incomplete in 24 (43%) cases. From the authors' personal experience left upper lobectomy was the most difficult, followed in order by right upper lobectomy, right middle lobectomy, and right lower lobectomy, with left lower lobectomy being the easiest.

Actual complications encountered were: (1) bleeding from a bronchial artery in one case during anterior-to posterior dissection of a bronchus. Bronchial arteries are often located posteriorly and cannot be seen if dissection proceeds only from anterior to posterior (Figs. 13.10c and 13.11a). Identifying and cauterizing bronchial arteries directly with the scope placed in the seventh (upper lobectomy) or eighth (lower lobectomy) intercostal space in the posterior axillary line (Figs. 13.10d and 13.11b), respectively, is the most reliable way to confirm hemostasis; (2) persistent air leakage in one case from a fissure sealed with LigaSure™ before we changed to using Enseal®, routinely. Chest tubes can be removed earlier when Enseal® is used compared with LigaSure™, because there is less air leakage when Enseal® is used during TPL. Thus, we prefer Enseal® for dividing thick lung parenchyma in an incomplete fissure in infants and children with small thoracic cavities when a 10 mm stapler is impractical; (3) bleeding due to a dislodged Hem-o-lok clip applied to a small thin A1+2, in one case. This case was treated by clipping both proximal and distal to the bleeding point and dividing between the proximal and distal clips with a pair of endoscopic scissors without LigaSure™ sealing. After the lung parenchyma in an incomplete fissure was divided with a stapler, there was blood in the fissure because of the dislodged clip. The clip was probably dislodged while using a stapler to complete the fissure. Because of this, we no longer clip small thin arteries; we seal the artery, confirm hemostasis, and then divide without clipping. For larger vessels, we only use clips proximally and always seal distally. While some surgeons use LigaSure™ for dividing all segmental pulmonary arteries, we prefer to apply a clip proximal to the point of division of a larger artery without clipping distally, and treat small thin arteries by sealing, purely to reduce the number of clips, so they do not obstruct the jaws of a stapler during application and firing.

If things are not progressing smoothly, never dissect from anterior to posterior under any circumstances. Add an extra trocar to improve visualization of all vital structures (Figs. 13.5d and 13.6b, c). From experience, the extra trocar is best placed in the posterior axillary line in the tenth intercostal space for a lower lobectomy and in the ninth intercostal space for an upper lobectomy. Switching the scope from the sixth intercostal space trocar to either the eighth or tenth intercostal space trocars during lower lobectomy and from the fifth intercostal space trocar to either the seventh or ninth intercostal space trocars during upper lobectomy greatly facilitates visualization and ensures safety (Figs. 13.5d and 13.6b, c).

## 13.10 In Closing

In all cases, the fundamental principles of TPL are the same, i.e., the surgeon should have in-depth knowledge of the anatomy of the pulmonary arteries, veins, and bronchi, including the various aberrant arteries/veins known to exist in each lobe, and also have confidence in treating incomplete fissures between lobes. If TPL seems too difficult, an extra trocar placed as described above will greatly facilitate safe completion of surgery.

## References

1. Rothenberg SS. Thoracoscopic lobectomy. In: Holcomb III GW, Georgeson KE, Rothenberg SS, editors. Atlas of pediatric laparoscopic and thoracoscopy. Philadelphia: Saunders, Elsevier; 2008. p. 253.
2. Stroedter L. Resection of pulmonary sequestrations. In: Saxena AK, Hollwarth ME, editors. Essentials of pediatric endoscopic surgery. Berlin: Springer; 2009. p. 105.
3. Polites SF, Habermann EB, Zarroug AE, et al. Thoracoscopic vs. open resection of congenital cystic lung disease—utilization and outcomes in 1120 children in the United States. J Pediatr Surg. 2016;51:1101–5.
4. Arai T, Shiozawa M. Pulmonary resections: anatomy and surgical technique. 2nd ed. Tokyo: Asakura; 2004. (In Japanese)
5. Koga H, Nakamura H, Murakami H, et al. Thoracoscopic Pulmonary Lobectomy for Densely Fused Pulmonary Lobes in Children with Congenital Pulmonary Airway Malformation: Technical Tips. J Laparoendosc Adv Surg Tech A. 2019;29:415–19.
6. Balsara KR, Balderson SS, D'Amico TA. Surgical techniques to avoid parenchymal injury during lung resection (Fissureless lobectomy). Thorac Surg Clin. 2010;20:365–9.
7. Sueyoshi R, Koga H, Suzuki K, et al. Surgical intervention for congenital pulmonary airway malformation (CPAM) patients with preoperative pneumonia and abscess formation: "open versus thoracoscopic lobectomy". Pediatr Surg Int. 2016;32:347–51.
8. Koga H, Suzuki K, Nishimura K, et al. Comparison of the value of tissue-sealing devices for thoracoscopic pulmonary lobectomy in small children: a first report. Pediatr Surg Int. 2014;30:937–40.
9. Yamataka A, Koga H, Ochi T, et al. Pulmonary lobectomy techniques in infants and children. Pediatr Surg Int. 2017;33:483–95.

# 14 Pathology of Congenital Cystic Lung Diseases

Mio Tanaka and Emi Takakuwa

**Abstract**

Congenital pulmonary airway malformation (CPAM) type 1, CPAM type 2, bronchial atresia, and intralobar and extralobar pulmonary sequestration (IPS/EPS) are congenital cystic lung diseases (CCLD) that are most frequently submitted for pathological examination, whereas lobar emphysema, CPAM type 4, and bronchogenic cyst are less common. CPAM type 0, CPAM type 3, and alveolar capillary dysplasia are extremely rare. Pulmonary interstitial emphysema is not actually congenital, but usually occurs in the neonatal period, and a differential diagnosis with CCLD is often required. Fetal lung interstitial tumor (FLIT) is a tumorous lesion that usually occurs in the neonatal period, and sometimes in the fetal period.

**Keywords**

Congenital cystic lung disease · Bronchogenic cyst · Bronchial atresia · Infantile lobar emphysema · Congenital pulmonary airway malformation · Intra/extralobar pulmonary sequestration · Pulmonary interstitial emphysema · Alveolar capillary dysplasia · Fetal lung interstitial tumor

## 14.1 Bronchogenic Cyst

Bronchogenic cyst (BC) is assumed to originate from supernumerary lung buds. It is most often found in the middle mediastinum and less frequently adjacent to the pulmonary hilus. Macroscopically, it is a unilocular mass containing mucinous substances (Fig. 14.1a, b), and it usually has no communication with the preexisting trachea, bronchus, or pulmonary parenchyma. The diameter of the cyst is approximately 4–5 cm, but sometimes exceeds 10 cm in older patients. Microscopically, the cystic wall is lined with ciliated columnar or pseudostratified columnar epithelium, and the walls contain cartilaginous islands, bronchial glands, or smooth muscle bundles, mimicking the structure of the normal bronchus (Fig. 14.1c). The epithelium sometimes shows squamous metaplasia. A differential diagnosis may be required from CPAM type 1 and esophageal duplication. However, BC can be distinguished from these diseases by its epithelial type on histology.

M. Tanaka (✉)
Department of Pathology, Kanagawa Children's Medical Center, Yokohama, Japan
e-mail: mio@zc4.so-net.ne.jp

E. Takakuwa
Department of Surgical Pathology, Hokkaido University Hospital, Sapporo, Japan



H. Sago et al. (eds.), *Congenital Cystic Lung Disease*, https://doi.org/10.1007/978-981-15-5175-8_14

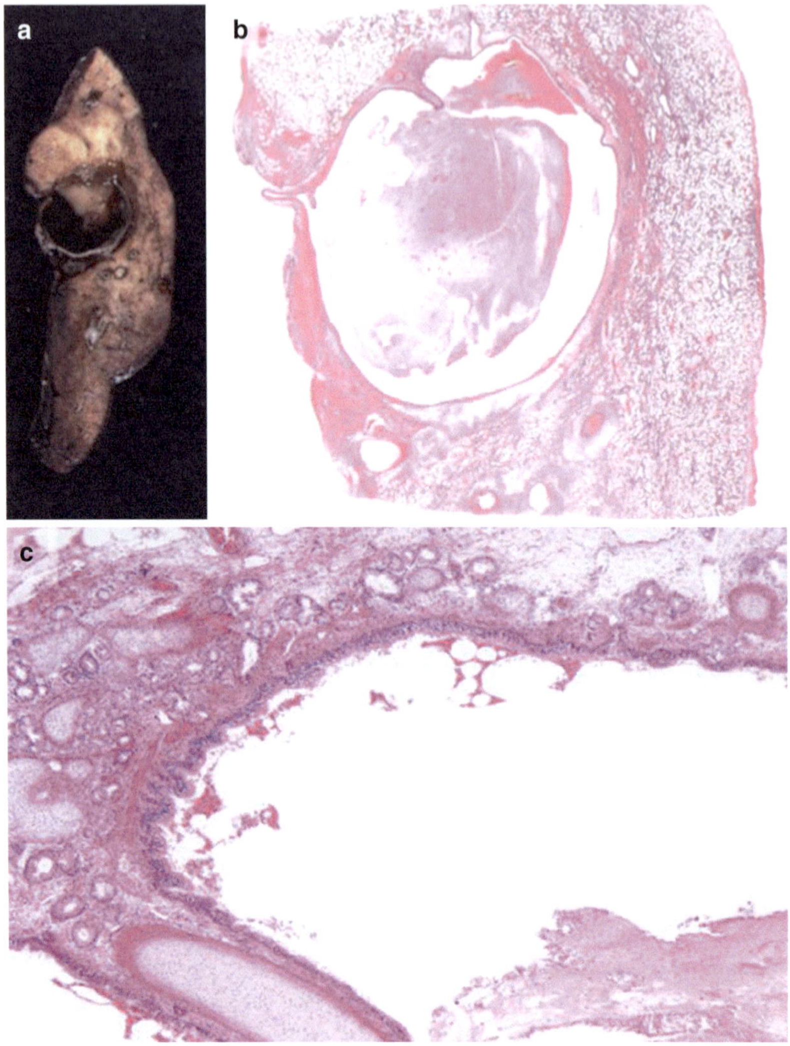

**Fig. 14.1** Bronchogenic cyst. (**a**, **b**) Macroscopic findings (**a**) and semi-macroscopic findings (**b**). A unilocular mass containing mucinous substances is present at the hilus. (**c**) Microscopic findings. The cystic wall is lined with ciliated columnar or pseudostratified columnar epithelium, and cartilaginous islands, bronchial glands, or smooth muscle bundles occur in the wall, mimicking the structure of the normal bronchus

## 14.2 Bronchial Atresia/Infantile Lobar Emphysema

### 14.2.1 Bronchial Atresia

Bronchial atresia (BA) is a relatively common CCLD, and is defined as a malformation of the pulmonary parenchyma resulting from atresia of the bronchus or bronchiole. Atresia of the bronchus is often detected in imaging studies before resection. On macroscopic examination, a mucus plug is seen at the atretic bronchus and cystic lesions around the atretic bronchus (Fig. 14.2a). The distal pulmonary parenchyma of the lesion is often emphysematous. Microscopically, a mucus plug is seen in the dilated bronchus and in the peripheral smaller bronchiole, which is diagnostic for BA (Fig. 14.2b, c). Fibrous tissues are seen at the atretic site, and the bronchial cartilage is often malformed. Variously sized cystic lesions lined with ciliated columnar epithelium, some of which have back-to-back bronchiole-like structures and are occasionally surrounded by smooth muscle bundles, are observed in the peripheral pulmonary parenchyma of the atretic bronchus (Fig. 14.2d). These findings are considered to indicate microcystic parenchymal maldevelopment of the bronchial atresia sequence [1]. The cystic lesions are similar to those of CPAM type 2. If distinct atresia of the bronchus is identified on macroscopic or micro-

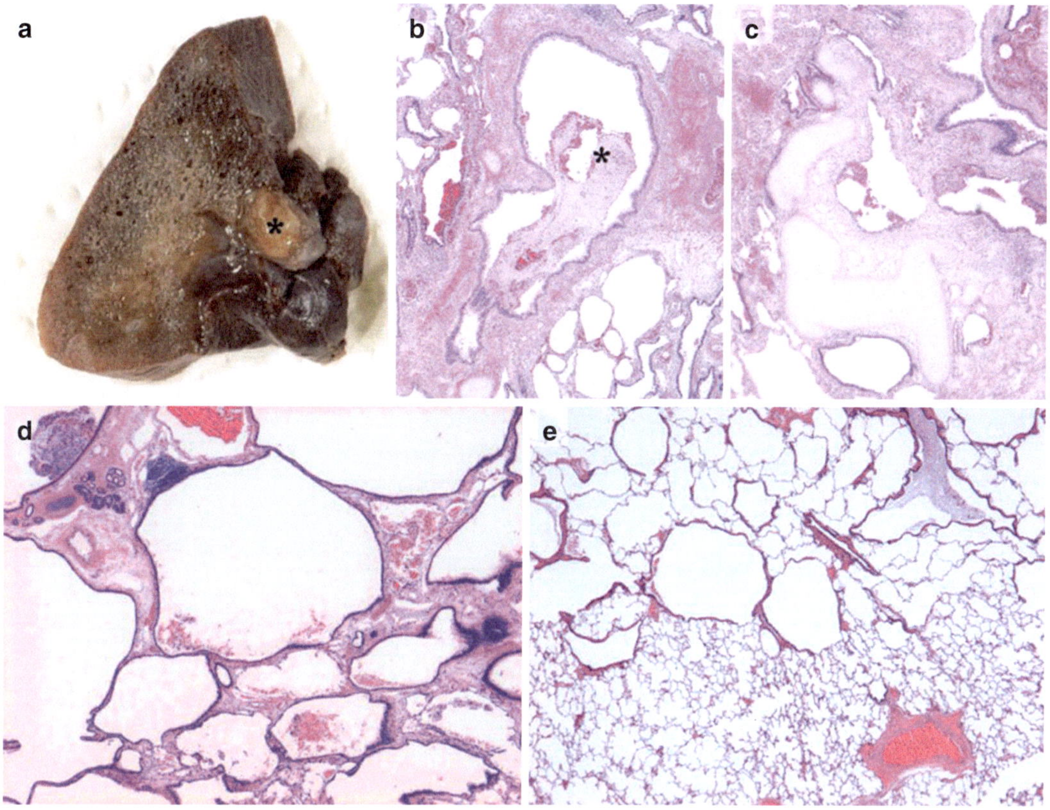


**Fig. 14.2** Bronchial atresia. (**a**) Macroscopic findings. A mucus plug is present at the atretic bronchus (asterisk), and small cystic lesions occur around the atretic bronchus. The distal pulmonary parenchyma is emphysematous. (**b**–**e**) Microscopic findings. A mucus plug is present in the dilated bronchus (asterisk, **b**). The cartilage around the atretic bronchus is often malformed (**c**). Variously sized cystic lesions lined with ciliated columnar epithelium, some with back-to-back bronchiole-like structures, known as microcystic parenchymal maldevelopment, occur around the atretic bronchus (**d**). The peripheral pulmonary parenchyma is emphysematous (**e**)

scopic examination, the lesion should be diagnosed solely as BA, and the term hybrid lesion of BA and CPAM type 2 should be avoided [2, 3]. Emphysematous changes are often observed around the lesions (Fig. 14.2e).

### 14.2.2 Infantile (Congenital) Lobar Emphysema (Overinflation)

Infantile lobar emphysema (ILE) is defined as the overinflation or hyperplasia of the pulmonary parenchyma associated with bronchial atresia or stenosis. It is attributed to a bronchial structural abnormality or extrinsic or intrinsic obstruction, although the cause of the atresia/stenosis is unclear in a considerable number of cases, even on histological examination. The lesion may involve the entire lobe or part of the lobe. On macroscopic examination, the affected lobe is hyperexpanded, and individual alveoli are sometimes visible (Fig. 14.3a). Microscopically, two patterns can be identified: the classic pattern and the hyperplastic (polyalveolar) pattern. In the classic pattern, the alveolar ducts and sacs are distended, often by as much as 3–10 times their normal size, and the alveolar walls are often focally disrupted (Fig. 14.3b, c). In the hyperplastic (polyalveolar) pattern, the lung parenchyma is more complicated, with an increased number of alveoli, and the radial alveolar counts are often 2–3 times that expected for the patient's age. The alveolar ducts and sacs may or may not be distended.

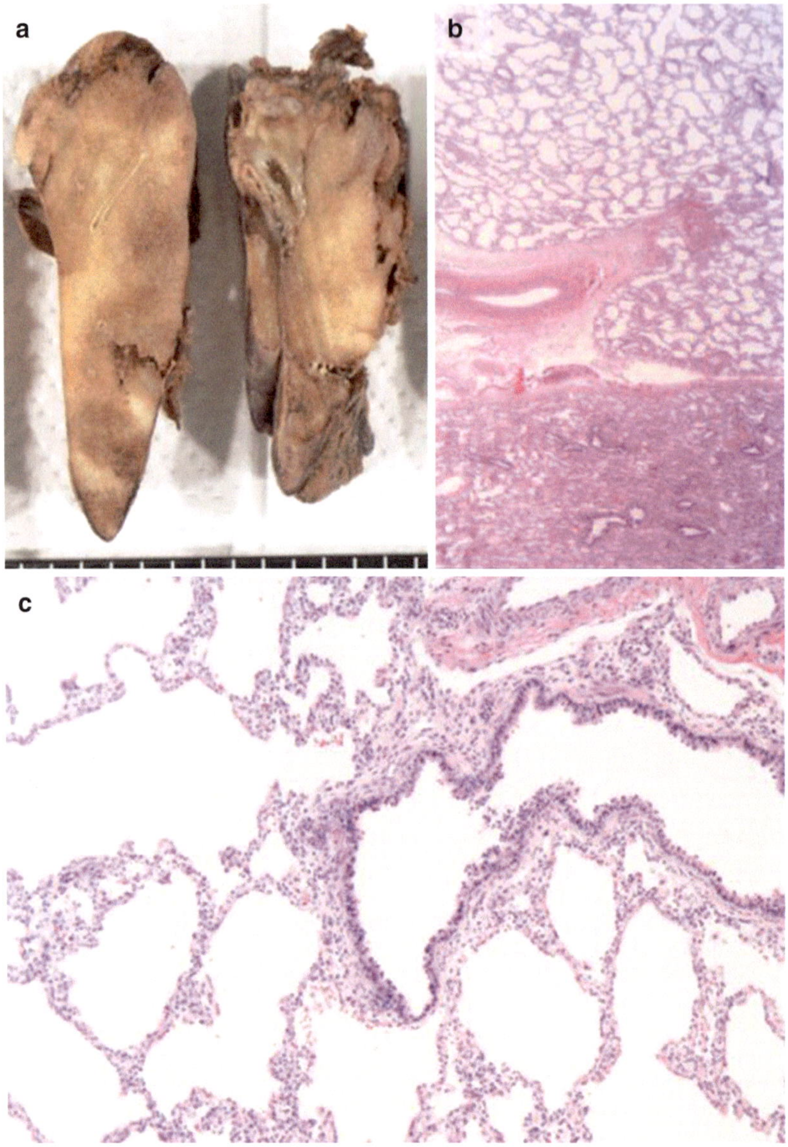

**Fig. 14.3** Lobar emphysema. (**a**) Macroscopic findings. The affected lobe is hyperexpanded. (**b**, **c**) Microscopic findings of the classic pattern. The alveolar ducts and sacs of the affected pulmonary parenchyma are distended (upper part of figure **b**) by up to 3–10 times the normal size. Lower part of (**b**) shows unaffected pulmonary parenchyma. The alveolar walls are often focally disrupted (**c**)

## 14.3 Congenital Pulmonary Airway Malformation

Congenital pulmonary airway malformation (CPAM) was originally described by Ch'In et al. in 1949 as a congenial cystic adenomatoid malformation (CCAM) [4]. In 1977, Stocker classified CCAM from type 1 to type 3, depending on the size of the cysts [5], and extended the classification to five types (types 0–4) based on the histological similarity of the cyst and airway structure of the trachea to alveoli, and introduced the term CPAM. CPAM is currently more commonly used than CCAM. In 2003, Langston established revised criteria for congenital cystic disease [1]. Further consideration of the definition of CPAM, including the clarification of its genetic background, is warranted.

### 14.3.1 CPAM Type 0

CPAM type 0, also described as congenital acinar dysplasia (CAD), is considered to arise from maturation arrest at the pseudoglandular stage, and is extremely rare and absolutely lethal. Macroscopically, the lesions are firm masses, and in cut section, show tiny scattered cystic lesions. Microscopically, the lesion is composed of bronchus-like structures without alveolar development, i.e., irregularly shaped tubules lined with simple or pseudostratified columnar epithelium, surrounded by mesenchymal tissues containing scattered muscle fibers, immature cartilaginous tissues, and large thin-walled vascular channels. Disruption of the TBX4–FGF10 pathway is reported to be a cause of CAD [6].

### 14.3.2 CPAM Type 1

CPAM type 1 was originally defined as a congenital cystic lesion composed of one or more large cysts, measuring more than 2 cm, with smaller cysts around the large cysts (Fig. 14.4a, b). It is reported to account for approximately 65% of all CPAMs [7]. Microscopically, the cysts are lined with ciliated columnar epithelium, often showing a sawtooth configuration. Clusters of mucogenic cells are present in the linings, surrounded by fibromuscular tissues, and in some cases, by malformed cartilage plates (Fig. 14.4c–e).

CPAM type 1 that undergoes surgical resection in the neonatal period may show smaller cysts (<2 cm). A rare type of CPAM type 1 composed only of small cysts, and the epithelium that

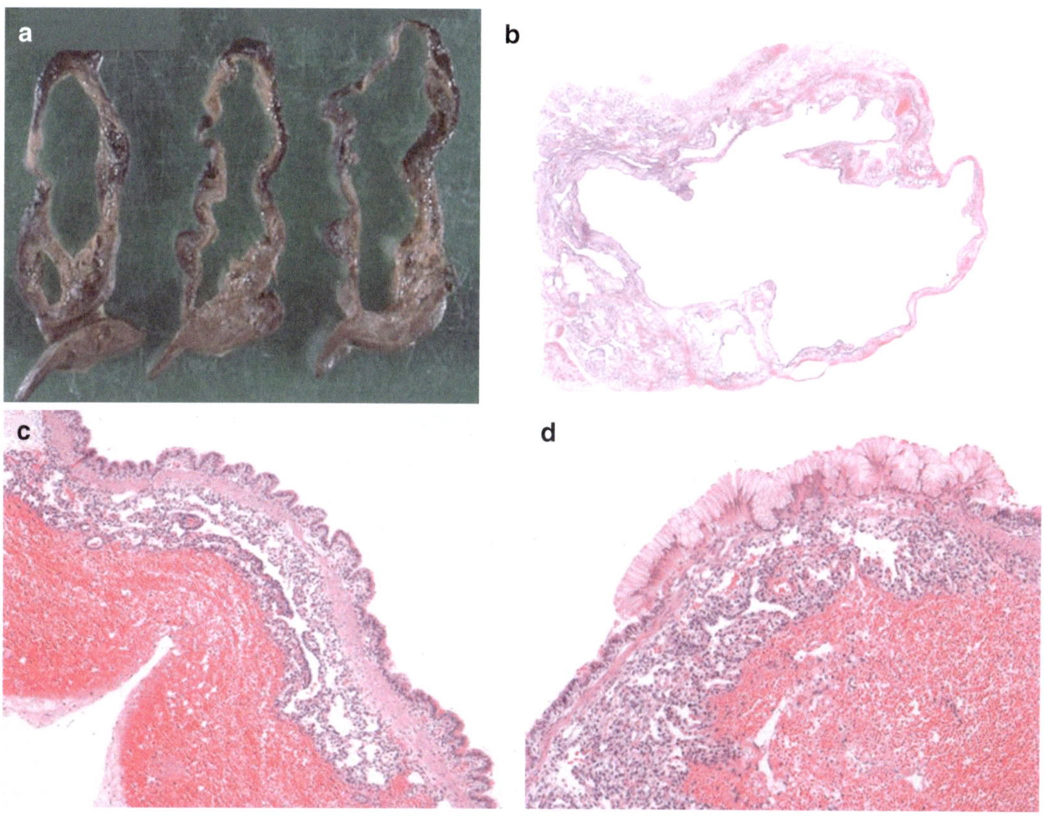


**Fig. 14.4** Congenital pulmonary airway malformation, type 1. (**a**, **b**) Macroscopic (**a**) and semi-macroscopic findings (**b**). The lesion is composed of one or more large cysts, with smaller cysts around the large cysts (**c**, **d**). Microscopic findings. The cysts are lined with ciliated columnar epithelium, often showing a sawtooth configuration (**c**), and clusters of mucogenic cells are present in the linings (**d**)

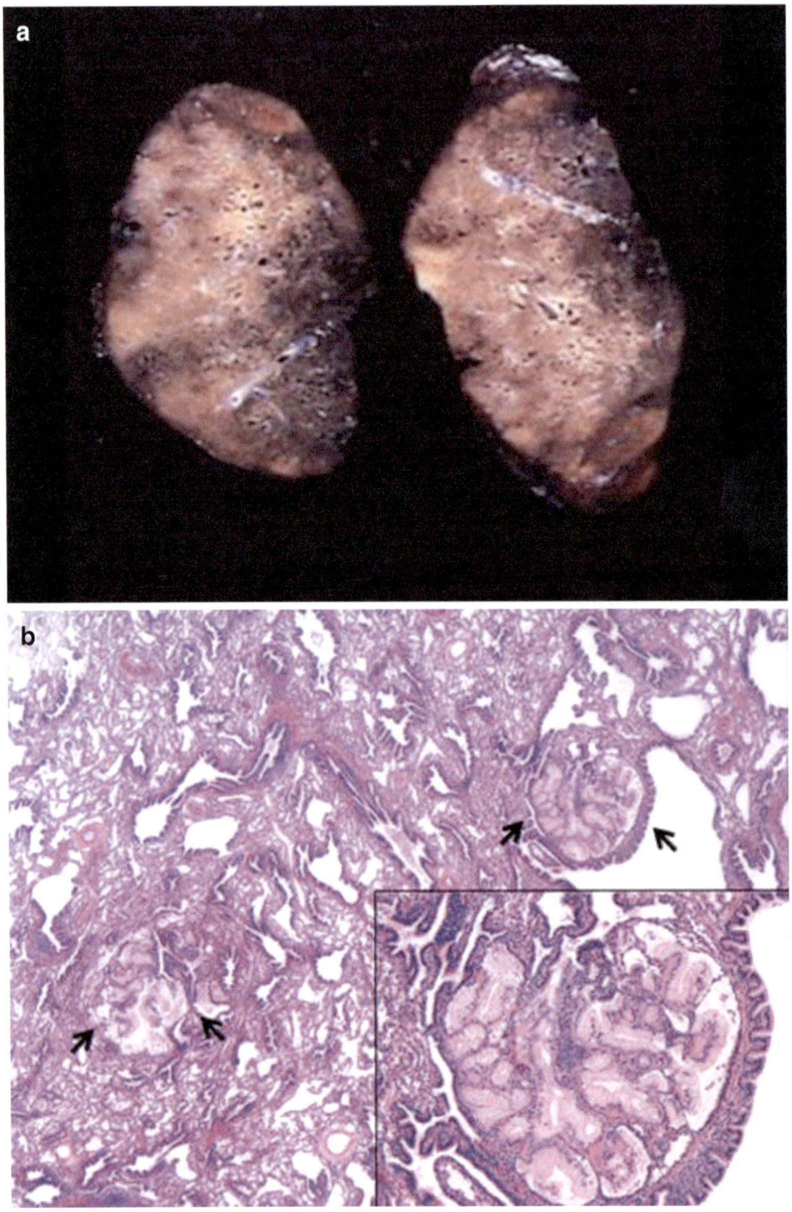

**Fig. 14.5** Congenital pulmonary airway malformation, type 1, solid variant. (**a**) Macroscopic findings. The cut surface is firm, with no large cyst, but scattered small cystic lesions are present. (**b**) Microscopic findings. The epithelium of the cysts are similar to those of classical CPAM type 1. Clusters of mucogenic cells are seen quite frequently in solid variants. Inset: high-power view of the cluster of mucogenic cells

is characteristic of CPAM type 1 (solid variant) is present (Fig. 14.5). Histological evidence of epithelium, particularly mucogenic cells, in addition to the size of the cyst are important for the diagnosis of CPAM type 1.

Some cases of CPAM type 1 were reported to develop into adenocarcinoma, usually in the form of bronchioloalveolar carcinoma, which is associated with the genetic background, including *KRAS* and *EGFR* mutations [8, 9].

### 14.3.3 CPAM Type 2

CPAM type 2 was originally defined as a congenital cystic lesion predominantly composed of uniformly sized cysts of <2 cm (Fig. 14.6a, b). It is reported to account for approximately 10–15% of CPAMs [7]. Microscopically, the cysts are lined with ciliated columnar epithelium, with back-to-back bronchiole-like structures, known as microcystic parenchymal maldevelopment,

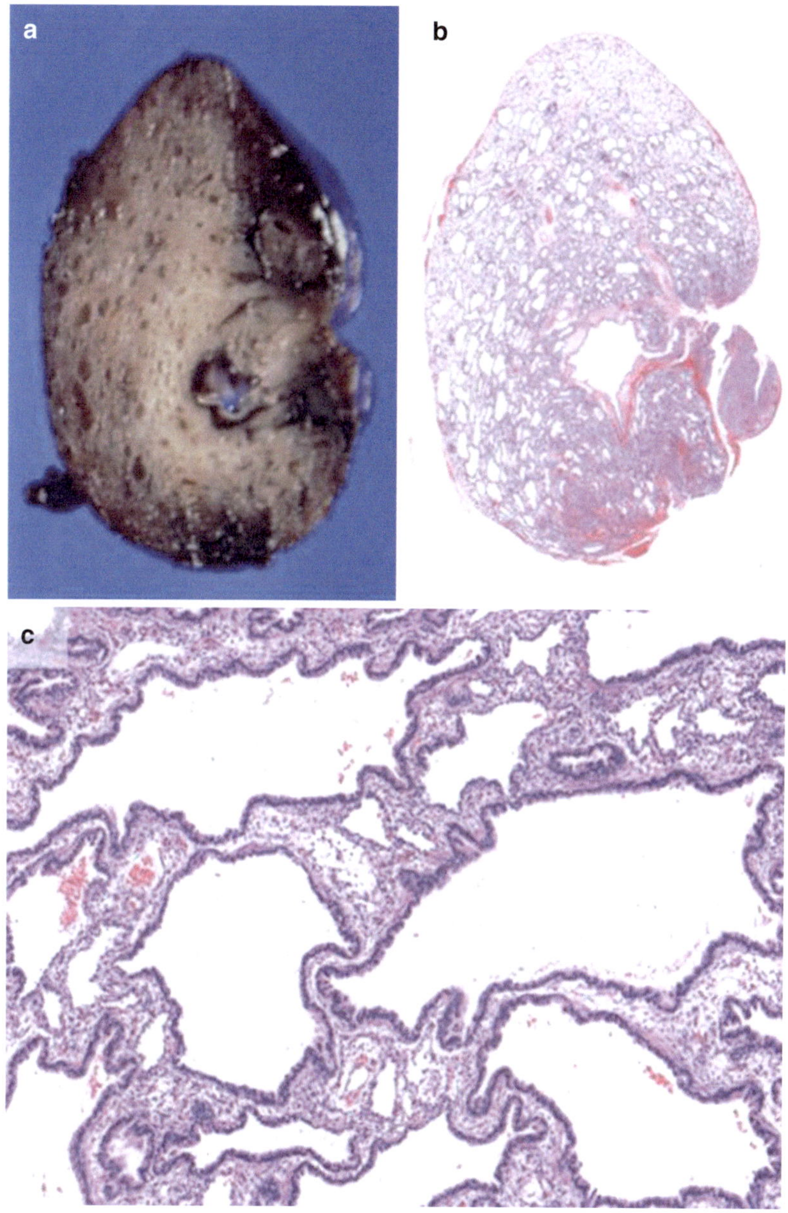


**Fig. 14.6** Congenital pulmonary airway malformation, type 2 (**a**, **b**). Macroscopic (**a**) and semi-macroscopic findings (**b**). The lesion is composed of predominantly uniformly sized cysts of <2 cm (**b**). Microscopic findings. The cysts are lined with ciliated columnar epithelium, and back-to-back bronchiole-like structures, occasionally surrounded by smooth muscle bundles, are observed (microcystic parenchymal maldevelopment). Normal alveolar structures and bronchioles are present in the lesions. No mucous plug is present (Courtesy of Dr. Yoshida, Hyogo Prefectural Kobe Children's Hospital)

and are occasionally surrounded by smooth muscle bundles (Fig. 14.6c). Normal alveolar structures and bronchioles are involved in the lesions. Mucogenic cells are not found in CPAM type 2. Rhabdomyoblasts are occasionally observed around the cysts (rhabdomyomatous dysplasia).

The histological findings are similar to those in the pulmonary parenchyma of bronchial atresia and pulmonary sequestration. Therefore, a diagnosis of CPAM type 2 should be avoided in patients in whom atresia of the bronchus or the presence of an aberrant artery is confirmed.

### 14.3.4 CPAM Type 3

CPAM type 3 is composed predominantly of uniformly sized cysts that rarely exceed 0.2 cm, and are firm solid lesions on macroscopic examination (Fig. 14.7a). CPAM type 3 involves the

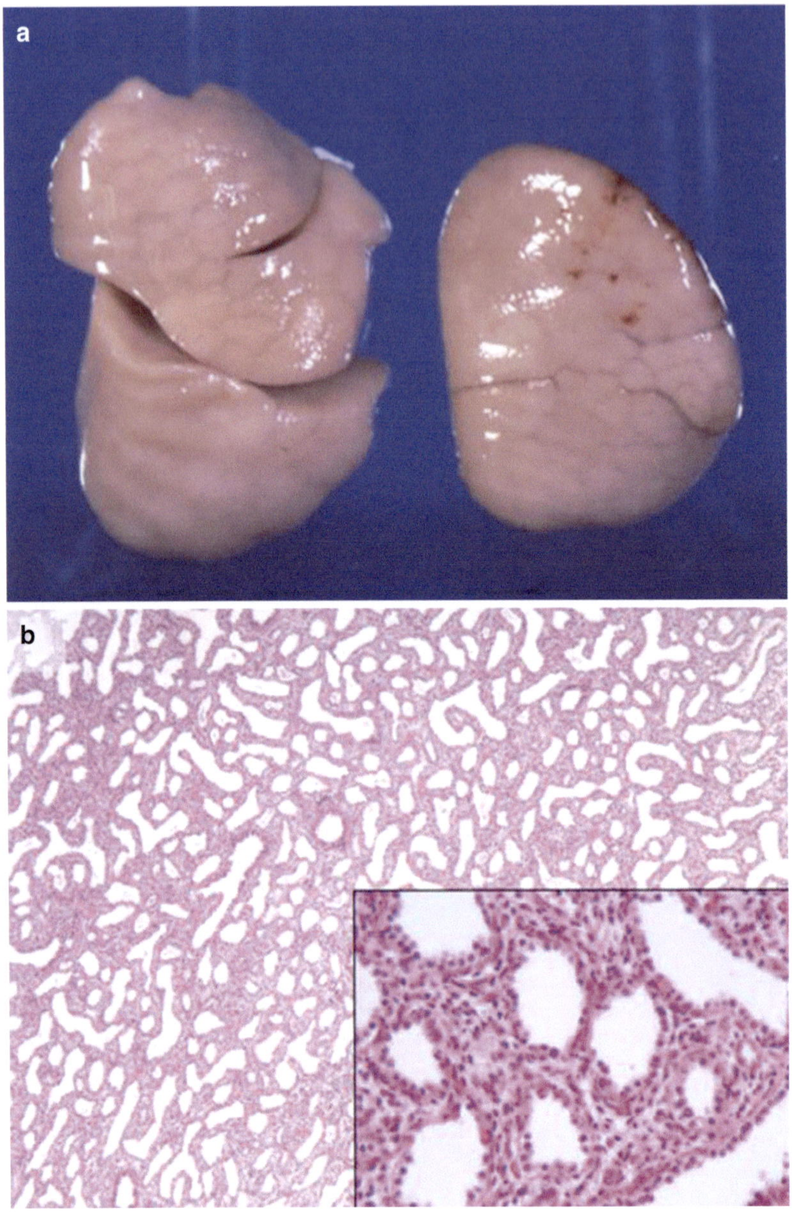


**Fig. 14.7** Congenital pulmonary airway malformation, type 3. (**a**) Macroscopic findings. The affected lung appears as a firm solid lesion. The entire lung of the presenting patient is affected. (**b**) Microscopic findings. The cysts resemble fetal lung tissue of the pseudoglandular period; evenly distributed small cysts lined with cuboidal epithelium, with no bronchial structure. Vessels are sparse. Inset: high-power view

entire lobe, or even the entire lung, and reportedly accounts for approximately 5% of all CPAMs [7]. Microscopically, the cysts resemble the fetal lung tissue of the pseudoglandular period, i.e., contain evenly distributed small cysts lined by cuboidal epithelium, with no bronchial structure (Fig. 14.7b). The septa are wider than in the normal fetal lung, and the vessels are sparse. Mucogenic cells and rhabdomyoblasts are not found in CPAM type 3.

### 14.3.5 CPAM Type 4

CPAM type 4 is usually located at the periphery of the lung, often beneath the pleura, and occasionally the lesion protrudes from the lung tissue (Fig. 14.8a). CPAM type 4 reportedly accounts for 10–15% of CPAMs [7]. On gross examination, the lesion is often composed of large cysts with thin septa. Microscopically, the cysts are lined with single flattened epithe-

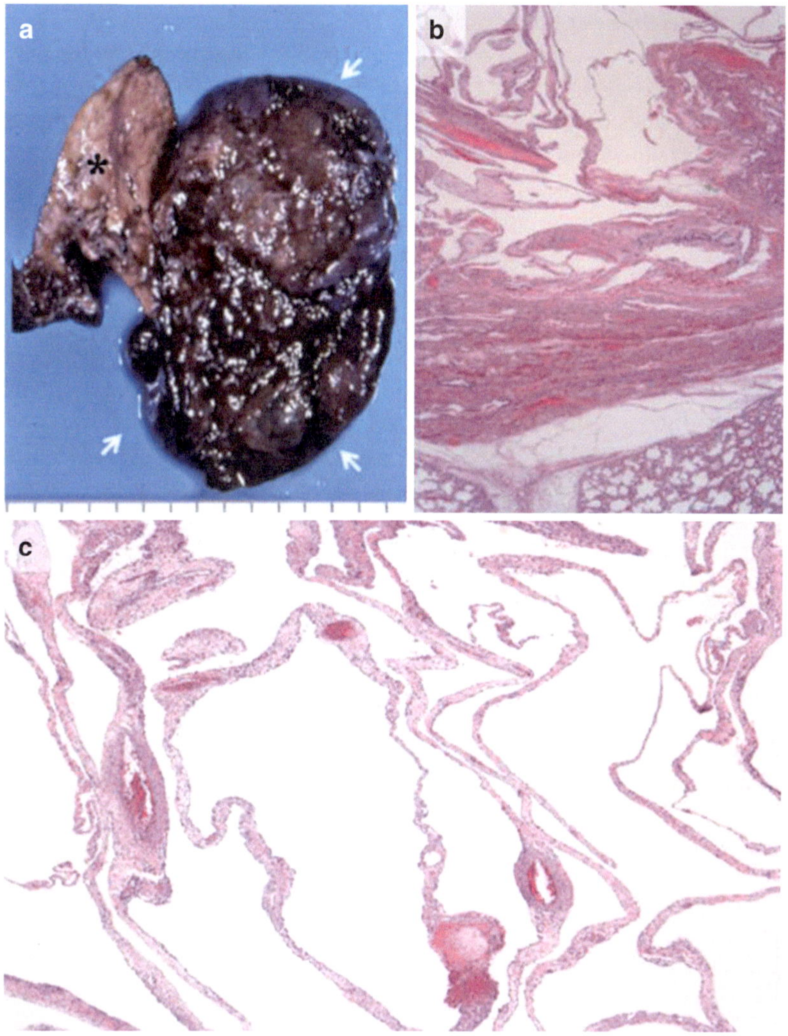


**Fig. 14.8** Congenital pulmonary airway malformation, type 4. (**a**) Macroscopic findings. The lesion is located at the periphery of the lung (arrow), and protrudes from the lung tissue (asterisk). (Courtesy of Dr. Matsuoka and Dr. Takeuchi, Osaka Women's and Children's Hospital). (**b**, **c**) Microscopic findings. The lesion is located beneath the pleura. Normal pulmonary parenchyma is seen in the lower part of (**b**). The lesion is composed of large cysts with thin septa, lined with single flattened epithelium resembling alveolar epithelium. No blastemal cells are present in the lesion

lium, resembling alveolar epithelium (Fig. 14.8b, c). CPAM type 4 and pleuropulmonary blastoma (PPB) type I (purely cystic PPB) are barely distinguishable from one another on imaging studies or gross examination. These lesions are known to be related by their background, as both involve an abnormality of the *DICER1* gene [10]. At the diagnosis of CPAM type 4, careful examination is required to detect the histological findings of PPB, such as a cluster of blastemal cells beneath the epithelium, described as cambium layer.

## 14.4 Sequestration

Pulmonary sequestration (PS) is defined as abnormal pulmonary tissue lacking any connection to the tracheobronchial tree, and has an anomalous systemic arterial supply. PS is considered to be a congenital malformation, possibly derived from a supernumerary lung bud. It is classified into two categories, intralobar and extralobar PS, depending upon its location in relation to the adjacent normal lung and its visceral pleural covering. Abnormal communication with the alimentary tract is observed in extremely rare cases.

### 14.4.1 Intralobar PS

Intralobar PS (IPS) is located within the lung tissue and lacks its own visceral pleura. It typically affects the lower lobes, most commonly in the left posterior basal segment. On gross inspection, an aberrant artery is present at the lower border of the pulmonary ligament, and the lymph nodes are often visible. On the cut surface, the sequestered segment of the lung shows variably sized cystic lesions or overinflation (Fig. 14.9a). Chronic inflammation is prominent in older children, but indistinct in infant patients. A dilated and tortuous aberrant artery is prominent in the sequestered segment (Fig. 14.9b). Microscopically, a large elastic artery occurs at the pulmonary ligament, and lymph nodes and a bronchus-like structure with bronchial cartilage and/or bronchial glands are seen adjacent to the artery (Fig. 14.9c–e).

The structure of the bronchial tree in a sequestered lung was investigated in a case series by Ishida et al., who demonstrated that "congenital" IPS showed the "peripheral type" structure, consisting of blind-ended bronchial trees running toward the insertion site of the aberrant elastic artery of the pulmonary ligament, and often accompanied by lymph nodes adjacent to the aberrant artery [11]. These three components, an aberrant elastic artery, blind-ended bronchus

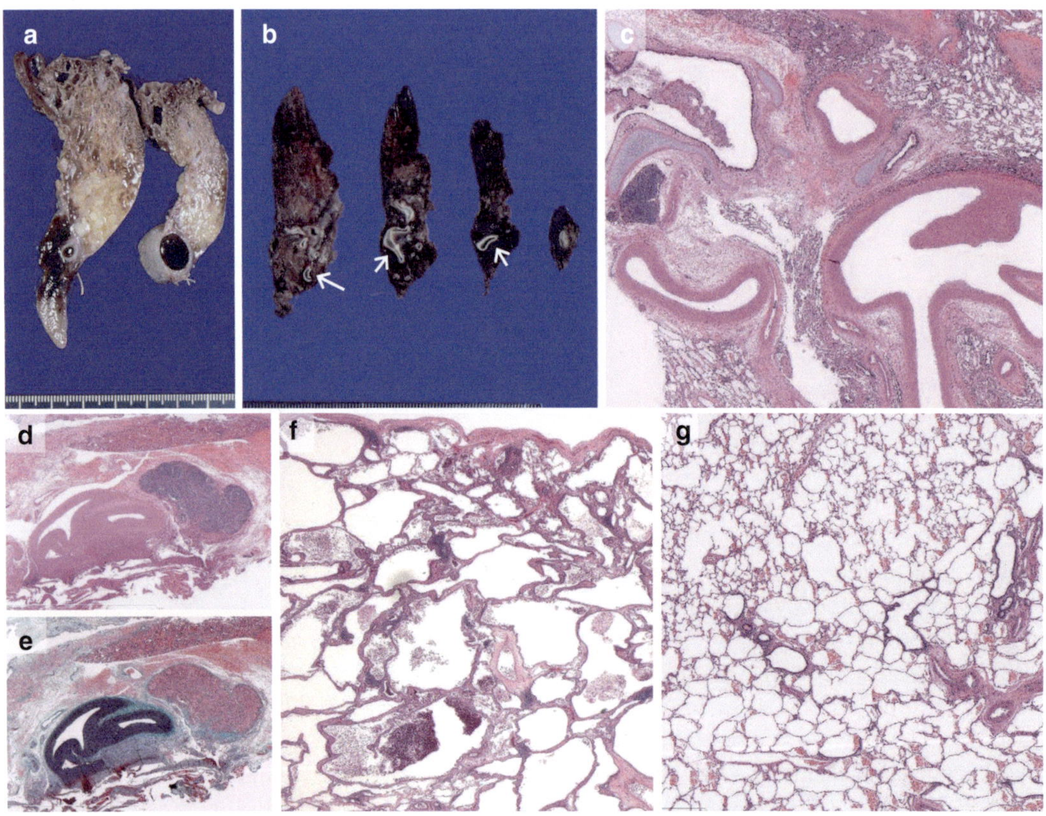

**Fig. 14.9** Intralobar pulmonary sequestration. (**a**, **b**) Macroscopic findings. Cystically dilated blind-ended bronchus and small cystic lesions with mucous retained in the parenchyma are present (**a**). At the cut surface, many anomalous vascular structures are present in the lower base segment (**b**, arrow). (**c**–**e**) Microscopic findings of aberrant hilus-like structures. Dilated bronchus with cartilage and bronchial glands (**c**), and Lymph node and aberrant elastic-type artery are present (**d**, **e**, **e**: Elastica Masson stain). (**f**, **g**) Microscopic findings of pulmonary parenchyma. The peripheral parenchyma shows microcystic maldevelopment, similar to CPAM type 2 (**f**), or hyperplasia-type maldevelopment (**g**)

with cartilage and/or bronchial glands, and lymph nodes, are regarded as ectopic hilus-like structures, and are the histological findings specific for congenital IPS.

IPS is considered to be a variant of bronchial atresia occurring in the posterior basal segment [1]. A parenchymal cystic lesion resembling CPAM type 2 is occasionally observed histologically (Fig. 14.9f, g), but it should not be diagnosed as a hybrid lesion of IPS and CPAM. The detection of an aberrant hilus-like structure is essential for a diagnosis of congenital IPS, and the aberrant artery must be an elastic artery. If the aberrant artery is a muscular artery, it should be regarded as a systemic–pulmonary shunt, which is usually associated with inflammatory changes.

### 14.4.2 Extralobar PS Without Foregut Communication

Extralobar PS (EPS) without foregut communication is a congenital anomaly, with its own pleural investment and separated from the normal lung parenchyma. On gross examination, EPS is an ovoid or pyramidal mass with a systemic arterial supply from the distal thoracic or proximal abdominal aorta, and venous outflow to the systemic veins. The cut surface reveals homogeneous lung parenchyma or a cluster of small cysts. Microscopically, a hilus-like structure is often seen near the cut surface (Fig. 14.10a, b). The parenchyma consists of dilated bronchioles, alveolar ducts, and alveoli, often containing mucous material and macro-

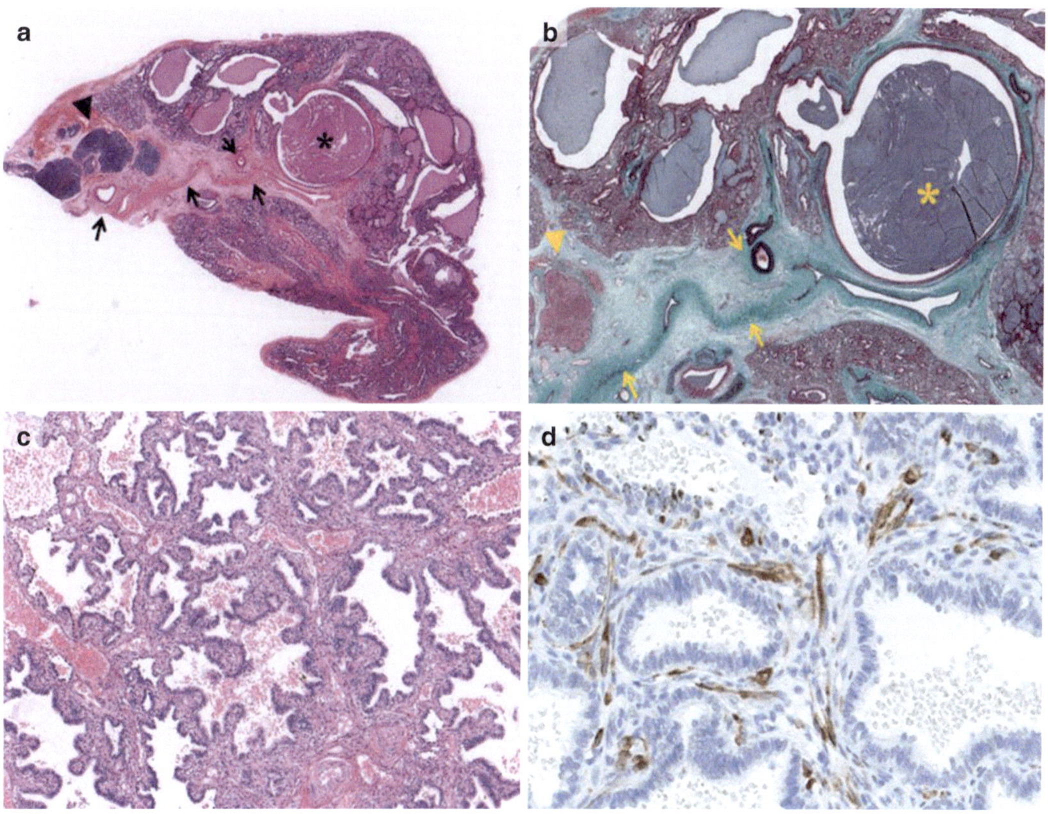


**Fig. 14.10** Extralobar sequestration. (**a–d**) Microscopic findings. Aberrant artery and vein (arrow), lymph node (arrowhead), blind-ended bronchus (asterisk), and small cysts with mucous retention are noted. (**a**, **b**, **b**: Elastica Masson stein). The parenchyma shows microcystic parenchymal maldevelopment (**c**). Desmin-positive striated muscle fibers are present in the cystic septum (**d**)

phages. An adenomatoid cystic lesion similar to that of CPAM type 2 is seen in about 50% of cases of EPS (Fig. 14.10c). Like IPS, these findings are considered to represent microcystic parenchymal maldevelopment of the bronchial atresia sequence, and EPS should not be diagnosed as a hybrid lesion of EPS and CPAM. In rare cases, striated muscle fibers in the cyst wall or around the alveoli are seen, described as rhabdomyomatous dysplasia (Fig. 14.10d).

### 14.4.3 Extralobar PS with Foregut Communication

Extralobar PS with foregut communication is an extremely rare congenital malformation, characterized by a communicating fistula between an isolated part of the respiratory system and the esophagus or stomach. The lining of the communicating fistula is ciliated or squamous epithelium.

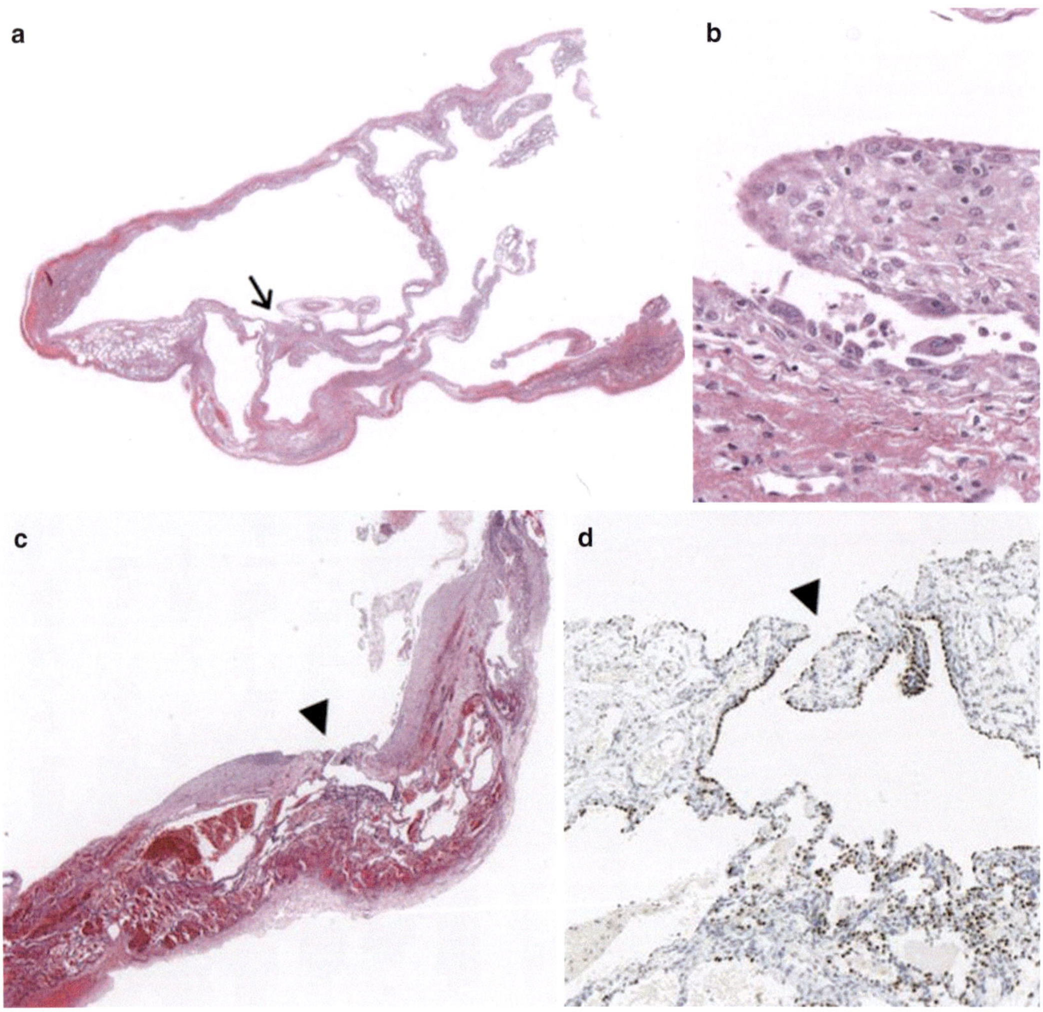


**Fig. 14.11** Pulmonary interstitial emphysema. (**a–d**) Microscopic findings. Large abnormal air spaces are present around the bronchovascular structure (**a**). Multinucleated foreign-body giant cells occur on the inner lumen of the air space, indicated with an arrow in figure **a** (**b**). Alveolar microcystic changes occur adjacent to the air spaces, and communication between the air spaces and the surrounding alveolar sacs can be seen (arrowhead). (**c**) TTF1-positive lining cells are continuous with the abnormal air space (**d**)

## 14.5 Pulmonary Interstitial Emphysema

Pulmonary interstitial emphysema (PIE) is defined as the dissection of bronchovascular structures and interlobular septa by air, and is usually associated with mechanical ventilation. PIE is an acquired lesion, but it is one of the most important differential diagnoses involving congenital cystic lung lesions in the neonatal period. PIE is classified as acute or persistent. On gross examination, PIE presents as air blebs of several millimeters on the pleural surface. Microscopically, the cysts are located in the interlobular septal and peribronchial regions. In persistent PIE, multinucleated foreign-body giant cells and many histiocytes line the abnormal space (Fig. 14.11a, b). Acute PIE lacks a histiocytic reaction and often communicates with the lymphatics of the interlobular area. Alveolar microcystic changes are occasionally seen at adjacent abnormal air spaces. The epithelial lining in the abnormal air space may be continuous with the alveolar cystic lesion (Fig. 14.11c, d).

## 14.6 Other Rare Diseases

### 14.6.1 Alveolar Capillary Dysplasia

Alveolar capillary dysplasia (ACD) is a rare and uniformly lethal disease, characterized by the maldevelopment of the alveolar capillaries. On macroscopic examination, the vessels may be prominent, but the macroscopic findings are otherwise unremarkable. Microscopically, the alveolar capillaries are relatively large, and are located in the center of the wide alveolar septa (Fig. 14.12a, b). Consequently, gas exchange at the alveoli is difficult. Misalignment of the pulmonary veins is commonly seen in ACD, and the pulmonary veins share the same adventia as the arteries (Fig. 14.12c, d).

The patient's condition is often complicated with other anomalies, such as congenital heart disease, urogenital anomalies, and gastrointestinal anomalies, and familial occurrence is also seen [12]. Deletions in the *FOX* gene and mutations in the *FOXF1* gene have been described as the causes of ACD [13].

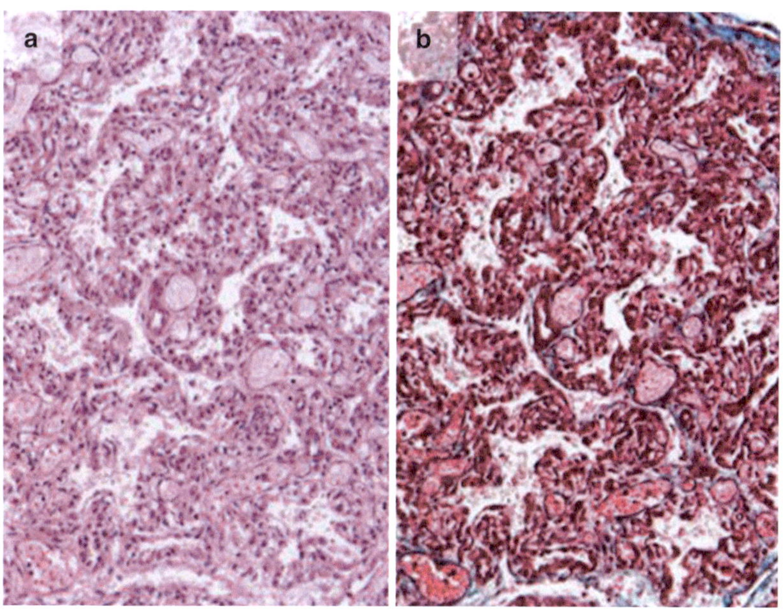


**Fig. 14.12** Alveolar capillary dysplasia. Microscopic findings. (**a**, **b**) Relatively large alveolar capillaries are located in the center of the wide alveolar septa. (**c**, **d**) Pulmonary vein shares the adventitia of the artery. (**b**, **d**) Elastica Masson stain

**Fig. 14.12** (continued)

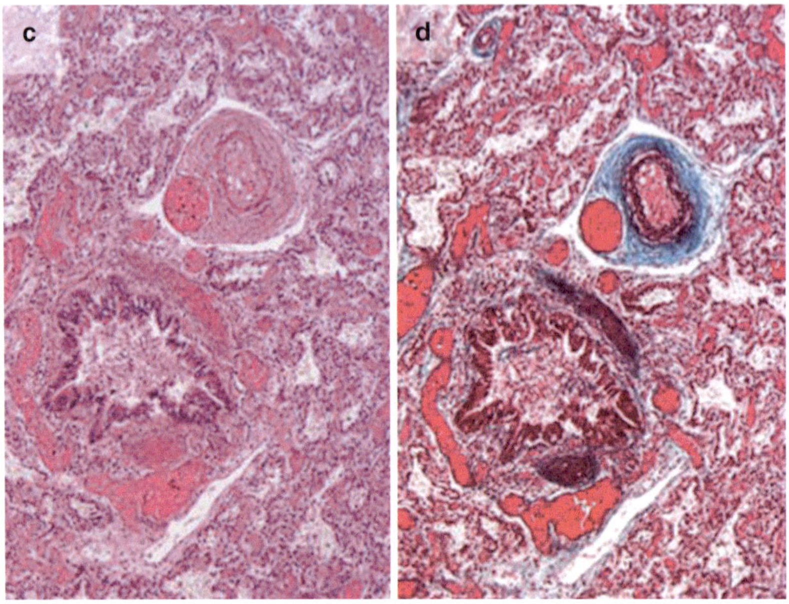


## 14.6.2 Fetal Lung Interstitial Tumor

Fetal lung interstitial tumor (FLIT) is a fetal intrapulmonary lesion newly characterized by Dishop et al. in 2010 [14], that usually develops in neonates or early infants. On macroscopic examination, FLIT presents as an intrapulmonary well-circumscribed solid mass (Fig. 14.13a). On microscopic examination, the lesion shows an immature alveola-like structure, resembling the fetal lung of the canalicular period (Fig. 14.13b). The alveola-like structure is lined with flattened or cuboidal epithelium without cilia. Scattered immature mesenchymal cells with round nuclei and abundant glycogen-rich cytoplasm within edematous stroma are present in the septa. No overt atypia is observed in either the epithelial or stromal cells. Small bronchus-like structures with smooth muscle bundles, immature cartilaginous tissues, and extramedullary hematopoiesis may occur in the lesion. The lesion has an incomplete fibrous capsule (Fig. 14.13c).

Chromosome 8 trisomy [15] and *ALK* rearrangement [16] are reported in cases of FLIT. Patients with *ALK* rearrangement may require a differential diagnosis with inflammatory myofibroblastic tumor [17]. The histological similarity of FLIT and CPAM type 3 has also been reported [18]. Further clarification of whether FLIT is developmental disorder or a true neoplastic lesion is required.

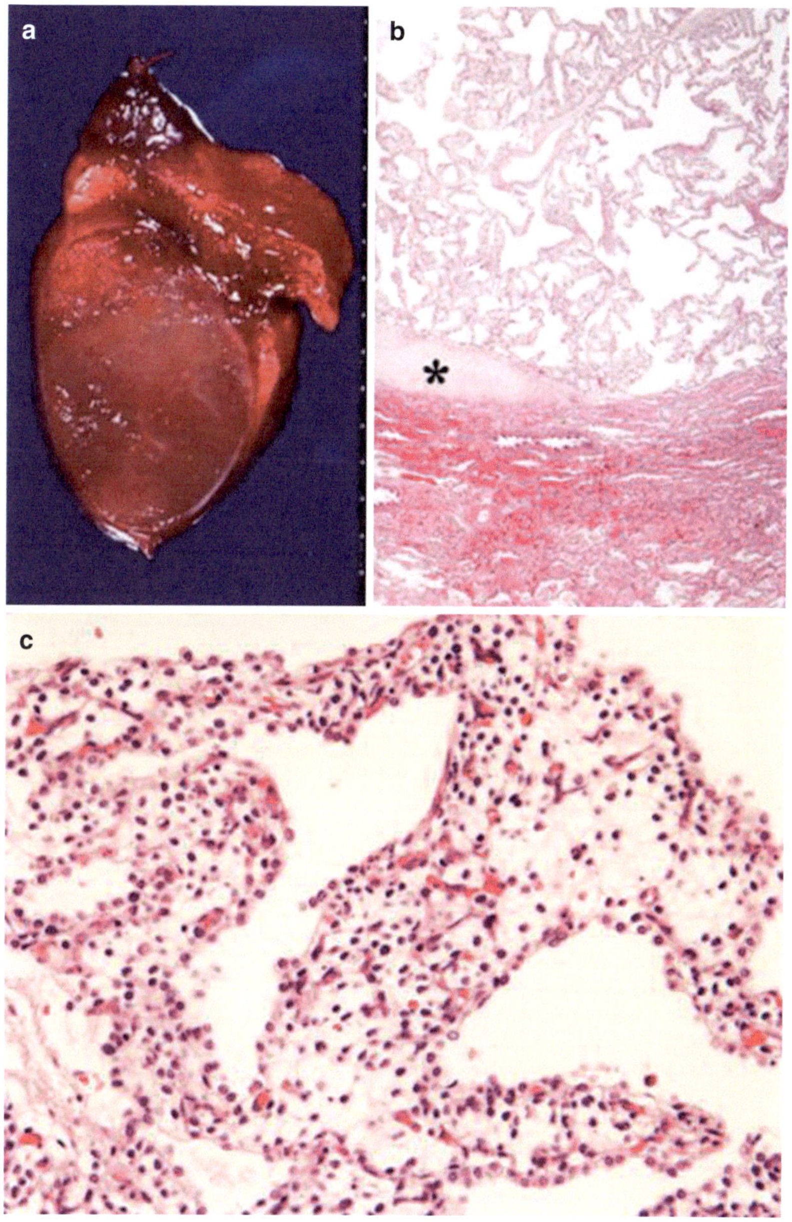


**Fig. 14.13** Fetal lung interstitial tumor. (**a**) Macroscopic findings. The lesion appears as an intrapulmonary well-circumscribed solid mass. (**b**, **c**) Microscopic findings. The lesion (upper part of the photo) has an incomplete fibrous capsule, containing immature cartilaginous tissue (asterisk, **b**). The lesion is composed of an immature alveola-like structure lined with flattened or cuboidal epithelium, without cilia. The septa contain scattered immature mesenchymal cells with round nuclei and abundant glycogen-rich cytoplasm within the edematous stroma (**c**)

## References

1. Langston C. New concepts in the pathology of congenital lung malformations. Semin Pediatr Surg. 2003;12:17–37.
2. Imai Y, Mark EJ. Cystic adenomatoid change is common to various forms of cystic lung diseases of children: a clinicopathologic analysis of 10 cases with emphasis on tracing the bronchial tree. Arch Pathol Lab Med. 2002;126:934–40.
3. Riedlinger WF, Vargas SO, Jennings RW, et al. Bronchial atresia is common to extralobar sequestration, intralobar sequestration, congenital cystic adenomatoid malformation, and lobar emphysema. Pediatr Dev Pathol. 2006;9:361–73.
4. Ch'In KY, Tang MY. Congenital adenomatoid malformation of one lobe of a lung with general anasarca. Arch Pathol. 1949;48:221–9.
5. Stocker JT, Madewell JE, Drake RM. Congenital cystic adenomatoid malformation of the lung. Classification and morphologic spectrum. Hum Pathol. 1977;8:155–71.
6. Karolak JA, Vincent M, Deutsch G, et al. Complex compound inheritance of lethal lung developmental disorders due to disruption of the TBX-FGF pathway. Am J Hum Genet. 2019;104:213–28.
7. Dehner LP, Stocker JT, Mani H, et al. Congenital pulmonary airway malformation in the respiratory tract. Philadelphia: Wolters Kluwer; 2016.
8. Guo H, Cajaiba MM, Borys D, et al. Expression of epidermal growth factor receptor, but not K-RAS mutations, is present in congenital cystic airway malformation/congenital pulmonary airway malformation. Hum Pathol. 2007;38:1772–8.
9. Lantuejoul S, Nicholson AG, Sartori G, et al. Mucinous cells in type 1 pulmonary congenital cystic adenomatoid malformation as mucinous bronchioloalveolar carcinoma precursors. Am J Surg Pathol. 2007;31:961–9.
10. Feinberg A, Hall NJ, Williams GM, et al. Can congenital pulmonary airway malformation be distinguished from type I pleuropulmonary blastoma based on clinical and radiological features? J Pediatr Surg. 2016;51:33–7.
11. Ishida H, Hajikano H, Hayashi A. Intralobal sequestration in children—a new concept from the form of bronchial tree in sequestrated lung. Nihon Kyobu Geka Gakkai Zasshi. 1992;40:957–68.
12. Slot E, Edel G, Cutz E, et al. Alveolar capillary dysplasia with misalignment of the pulmonary veins: clinical, histological, and genetic aspects. Pulm Circ. 2018;8:2045894018795143.
13. Stankiewicz P, Sen P, Bhatt SS, et al. Genomic and genic deletions of the FOX gene cluster on 16q24.1 and inactivating mutations of FOXF1 cause alveolar capillary dysplasia and other malformations. Am J Hum Genet. 2009;84:780–91.
14. Dishop MK, McKay EM, Kreiger PA, et al. Fetal lung interstitial tumor (FLIT): a proposed newly recognized lung tumor of infancy to be differentiated from cystic pleuropulmonary blastoma and other developmental pulmonary lesions. Am J Surg Pathol. 2010;34:1762–72.
15. de Chadarevian JP, Liu J, Pezanowski D, et al. Diagnosis of "fetal lung interstitial tumor" requires a FISH negative for trisomies 8 and 2. Am J Surg Pathol. 2011;35:1085. author reply 1086–1087
16. Onoda T, Kanno M, Sato H, et al. Identification of novel ALK rearrangement A2M-ALK in a neonate with fetal lung interstitial tumor. Genes Chromosomes Cancer. 2014;53:865–74.
17. Tanaka M, Kohashi K, Kushitani K, et al. Inflammatory myofibroblastic tumors of the lung carrying a chimeric A2M-ALK gene: report of 2 infantile cases and review of the differential diagnosis of infantile pulmonary lesions. Hum Pathol. 2017;66:177–82.
18. Yoshida M, Tanaka M, Gomi K, et al. Fetal lung interstitial tumor: the first Japanese case report and a comparison with fetal lung tissue and congenital cystic adenomatoid malformation/congenital pulmonary airway malformation type 3. Pathol Int. 2013;63:506–9.

# The Long-Term Outcome of Congenital Cystic Lung Disease

# 15

Yuko Tazuke

**Abstract**

Advances in neonatal care have improved the survival rate of patients with CCAM, and the postoperative long-term follow-up have become more important for CCAM patients. This chapter describes the long-term outcome, including chest deformity, scoliosis, the respiratory function, and pulmonary complications. The thoracic deformity or scoliosis might be worse during the growth period. And some cases have risk of pulmonary complications, as pneumonia, pneumothorax, and cancer, while, the clinical course of lung function during adolescence and adulthood is still unclear. The careful follow-up is necessary for CCAM cases in which surgical intervention is difficult and in asymptomatic CCAM cases.

**Keywords**

Congenital cystic lung disease · Long-term outcome · Long-term complications · Thorax deformation · Scoliosis · Respiratory functions · Malignancy

Congenital pulmonary airway malformation (CPAM), previously known as congenital cystic adenomatoid malformation (CCAM), is a developmental lesion of the lung composed of single or multiple cysts of uniform or varying sizes arising from anomalous growth of the airways. Because CPAM can cause pulmonary hypoplasia, severe nonimmune fetal hydrops, and fetal death [1–6], most studies have focused on the short-term outcome of CCAM diagnosed in the fetal period.

In a Japanese nationwide multicentric study, most early operative cases involved in infants and neonates with acute respiratory distress due to pulmonary hypoplasia [7]. However, patients with CCAM present with various symptoms that range from acute respiratory distress due to pulmonary hypoplasia to mild ventilatory impairment and late-onset recurrent infection, with some patients remaining asymptomatic until adulthood. Recently, advances in neonatal care have improved the survival rate of patients with CCAM, and the different clinical courses of CCAM and postoperative long-term follow-up have become more important.

This chapter describes the long-term outcome, including chest deformity, scoliosis, the respiratory function, and pulmonary complications.

Y. Tazuke (✉)
Department of Pediatric Surgery, Osaka University Graduate School of Medicine, Osaka, Japan
e-mail: tazuke@pedsurg.med.osaka-u.ac.jp



H. Sago et al. (eds.), *Congenital Cystic Lung Disease*, https://doi.org/10.1007/978-981-15-5175-8_15

## 15.1 Thorax Deformation and Scoliosis

Factors that affect chest deformity and scoliosis may include the operative period, the operation method, and other non-operation-related factors. Although there have been some reports about the association of the operation method with the complication of thorax deformation [8], few studies have investigated the association between the operative period and the appearance of thorax deformation. Even if there are no findings on postoperative neonatal X-ray examination, chest deformity may appear at school age (Fig. 15.1). In patients who have undergone thoracotomy, including neonatal surgery cases, the thoracic deformity may shift to scoliosis during the growth period and follow-up is necessary. Minimally invasive surgery has emerged as the standard of care for many pediatric surgical conditions [8]. The stated advantages over standard thoracotomy include better postoperative pain control, a shorter hospital stay, and improved cosmesis.

Lu et al. reported that thoracoscopic resection of CCAM is associated with a longer operative time, shorter hospital stay, and potentially reduced complications, with no additional costs, with the main risk factor for conversion to thoracotomy being a past history of pneumonia [9]. With the increasing use of video-assisted thoracoscopic surgery (VATS), thoracoscopic resection of cystic lesions may well become the future standard of care for asymptomatic CCAM in children.

Taiwo et al. [10] examined the mid-term musculoskeletal status of patients who underwent VATS in comparison to those who underwent conventional thoracic surgery (CTS). The difference between the mean maximum range of motion of the shoulder joint on the operated and non-operated sides in the VATS and CTS groups did not differ to a statistically significant extent for any of the movements that were assessed. It is noteworthy that grade I scoliosis was observed in three patients who underwent VATS (9.7%) and 14 patients (53.8%) who underwent CTS ($p < 0.001$), although none of the patients developed grade II (moderate) or III (severe) scoliosis.

In our experience (Table 15.1), chest deformity was observed in 80% of patients who underwent early/emergency surgery and in 40% of the patients who underwent elective surgery. The frequency of chest deformity was high in the early surgery group. One of the reasons for this was the difference in surgery methods. Especially in recent years, thoracoscopic surgery has come to be performed in the standby surgery group. Based on the fact that thoracic deformity was not observed in three patients in the elective operation group who underwent thoracoscopic surgery, the introduction of thoracoscopic surgery seems have the potential to reduce the incidence of thoracic deformity as a long-term outcome.

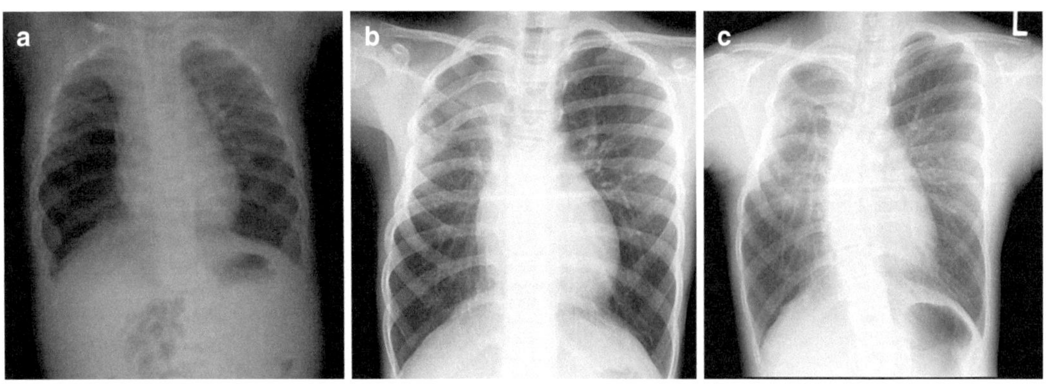


**Fig. 15.1** A series of X-ray findings after operation of right side of CCAM. Chest deformity may appear at school age. (**a**) 1 year after operation, (**b**) 8 years old, (**c**) 17 years old

**Table 15.1** Thorax deformation and scoliosis in our institutional study

| | Emergency surgery ($N = 21$) | Elective surgery ($N = 19$) | $p$ |
|---|---|---|---|
| Postoperative observation period (years) | 13 (0–26) | 4 (1–20) | <0.01 |
| Chest deformity | 76% (16/21) | 42% (8/19) | 0.06 |
| Fusion of ribs or narrowing intercostal spaces | 62% (13/21) | 11% (82/19) | <0.01 |
| Scoliosis | 19% (4/21) | 5% (1/19) | 0.35 |
| Pectus excavatum | 24% (5/21) | 21% (4/19) | 0.57 |
| Operative case for pectus excavatum | 2/5 | 0/4 | |
| Asthma | 14% (3/21) | 21% (4/19) | 0.69 |

## 15.2 Pectus Excavatum

Tainaka et al. [11] showed there was no significant difference in the incidence of pectus excavatum at complete thoracoscopic lobectomy for congenital cystic lung disease between neonatal and infantile patients (neonates vs. infants: 7.1% vs. 4.2%, $p = 1.00$). In our study (see Table 15.1), the incidence of funnel chest did not differ between the emergency surgery group and elective surgery group. However, symptoms may appear with the growth of the body, and the continuous follow-up of these patients is necessary (Fig. 15.2).

Long-term complications, including such as conventional thoracic deformity, are expected to be improved in cases asymptomatic CCAM, bronchial atresia or pulmonary sequestration in which it is possible to perform elective surgery using VATS.

## 15.3 The Respiratory Function

There are only a limited number of longitudinal studies on the pulmonary function of patients with a history of CCAM. Barikbin et al. [12] performed postoperative lung function tests to assess

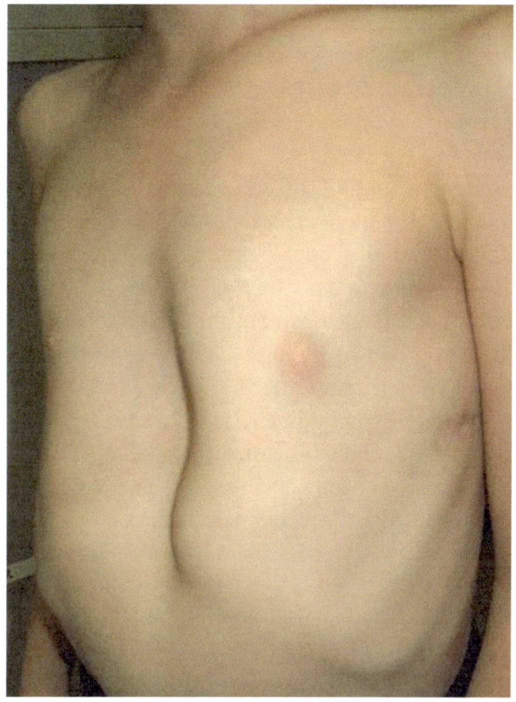

**Fig. 15.2** Pectus excavatum

26 CCAM patients (median age 15.5 years; range, 6–45 years) and compared the results to those of healthy patients (controls, median age 10 years; range, 1–61 years). The CCAM patients showed restrictive ventilation disorder with increased respiratory rates ($p = 0.006$) and marginally decreased tidal volumes ($p = 0.043$). Furthermore, respiratory compliance was significantly reduced in comparison to controls ($p < 0.001$). Although no statistically significant differences were seen in the respiratory resistance, functional residual capacity, or capillary blood gas levels, the postoperative respiratory compliance was significantly recovered ($p < 0.001$) in the CCAM infants who underwent surgery in the first 2 years of life. Frenckner et al. [13] found a very mild reduction of vital capacity, total lung capacity, and forced expiratory volume in one second (FEV1) in children at 7 years (mean) after surgery, while the FRC value was slightly higher than the predicted value for age. Keijzer et al. [14] compared the lung function in school age children after early (<2 years) and late (>2 years) lobectomy. Both groups showed a

mild impairment in forced vital capacity and FEV1 without statistically significant differences between early and late resection. Spoel et al. [15] measured the lung function of infants with congenital lung lesions, including CCAM, who underwent surgery at 6 and 12 months of age and reported that surgical resection did not negatively affect the clinical course or lung function.

According to our experience (Table 15.1), the history of asthma treatment did not differ between the two groups. Although, there was no correlation between chest deformity and the current respiratory symptoms, the long-term respiratory symptoms and the time of surgery, a larger number of cases is needed before any statistically significant differences can be determined.

Moreover, patients who require long-term ventilatory support, including those with severe CCAM, are at risk of developing bronchopulmonary dysplasia (BPD). BPD is the most common form of chronic lung disease in infancy. The disease was seen in large preterm infants with severe respiratory distress syndrome who had been treated with high inspired oxygen concentrations and prolonged mechanical ventilation with high positive airway pressure resulting in inflammation, fibrosis, and smooth muscle hypertrophy in the airways [16]. There have only been a limited number of longitudinal studies on the pulmonary function of patients with a history of BPD. Blayney et al. [17] investigated children with BPD at 7 and 10 years of age (mean ages) and found an improvement in the forced expiratory volume in one second over time in a subgroup of patients with abnormal values at 7 years of age. This might suggest that continuing lung growth and repair occurs in school-aged children [18]. Koumbaroi et al. [19] followed patients with chronic lung disease with annual measurements of the pulmonary function from 8 years of age to 15 years of age (mean age). In patients with mild chronic lung disease, air trapping gradually normalized; however, half of the patients had abnormal spirometric values indicating small airway obstruction. The clinical course of lung function during adolescence and adulthood is currently unclear due to a lack of relevant longitudinal studies [18].

## 15.4 Developmental Assessment

There have been no reports on long-term developmental and neurological assessment in CCAM. However, extracorporeal membrane oxygenation (ECMO) has been used for the management of CCAM neonates with severe cardiopulmonary failure who fail to respond to conventional therapy [20, 21]. Jsselstijn et al. [22] describe some developmental problems as long-term outcomes of children treated with neonatal extracorporeal membrane oxygenation. As they become older, most patients—except those with congenital diaphragmatic hernia (CDH)—have a normal lung function and normal growth. The maximal exercise capacity is below normal and seems to deteriorate over time in the CDH population. Gross motor function problems have been reported until school age. Although mental development is usually favorable within the first years and cognition is normal at school age, many children experience problems with working speed, spatial ability tasks, and memory. Thus, they concluded that because children who survived neonatal treatment with ECMO often encounter neurodevelopmental problems in school age, long-term follow-up is needed to recognize problems early and to offer appropriate intervention [22].

## 15.5 Pneumonia and Other Complications

Ten to forty percent of patients with CPAM will develop significant pulmonary infections [23, 24], and cases of malignant lesions associated with CPAM have also been reported [25, 26]. Survey data from a study with a median follow-up period of 3.9 years (range, 0.2–13.2 years) revealed that 17% of patients with CPAM developed chronic pulmonary symptoms, including cough (11%) and asthma requiring bronchodilator therapy (12%) [27].

Enuh et al. reported CPAM with aspergillosis in a 59-year-old man who died secondarily to massive hemoptysis and the development of disseminated intravascular coagulation during lobectomy [28]. Morelli et al. reported a case of CPAM involving a 38-year-old man with persistent cough and hemoptysis, who did well after lobectomy [29]. In adults, CPAM appears as a large cyst or a cluster of cysts filled with gas or liquid resembling a solid mass in CT scans [30]. Because of the higher percentage of asymptomatic cases of CPAM and the various degrees of lung involvement, it might be difficult to determine the prognosis in adults [31]. A meta-analysis of the postoperative management of congenital cystic lung lesions showed that elective surgery is associated with better outcomes than emergency surgery; however, the risk of symptoms occurring in previously asymptomatic cases is small [32]. In their retrospective review of 81 patients, Fascetti-Leon et al. found lung sparing resection to be safe and effective with no increased risk of residual disease or recurrence if accurately planned in selected patients [33].

## 15.6 Pneumothorax

The risk of recurrent pneumothorax or infectious complications is unknown due to the limited published information on the long-term outcomes or complications in patients with resected CPAM lesions. However, Shupe et al. [34] described a case in which isolated spontaneous pneumothorax occurred as a long-term complication of CPAM in an adult patient who had undergone neonatal lobectomy. Such cases have residual disease and moderate fixed obstructive/restrictive defects are observed on lung function testing.

On rare occasions, CPAM can present in adulthood with recurrent chest infections, pneumothorax, hemoptysis, or dyspnea [35, 36]. Hamanaka et al. [37] reviewed 61 adult cases of CCAM reported in the literature, and 7 of the patients (11.7%) presented with pneumothorax, while 21 (35%) presented with infection. The follow-up of all CPAM patients should include an evaluation for evidence of residual lung disease both with spirometric testing and chest imaging. Furthermore, physicians should be aware of the possibility of infectious complications and symptomatic obstructive lung disease.

## 15.7 Malignancy

Cases of malignancy emerging from CPAM have been described in several literatures.

In 2005 Laberge et al. [38] found five published cases of pleuropneumonary blastoma (PPB), seven cases of rhabdomyosarcoma, and eight cases of bronchioloalveolar carcinoma associated with CCAM lesions. Hartman et al. reported that 4% of pulmonary tumors were associated with congenital cystic malformations [39]. Nasr et al. revealed that the incidence of PPB in patients with preexisting suspected CPAM was 2% [40]. Papagiannopoulos et al. reported the cases of seven patients who were diagnosed with pulmonary cystic lesions and who later developed PPB in the same lung region. All of these patients underwent surgical resection after being diagnosed with CPAM. In six of the seven patients, the tumor developed in the area of the cysts [41].

A systematic review by Casangre et al. analyzed CPAM-associated lung tumor cases in children and adults. They could not find any age limit for malignant progression or definitive order for the malignant transformation of CPAM. The evolution of CPAM is unpredictable as there was no specific time delay between the diagnosis of CPAM and the emergence of a tumor [42].

Recently, PPB has been recognized as part of the spectrum of DICER1 mutation-related tumors, including sex cord stromal tumors, medulloepithelioma, thyroid carcinoma, and cystic nephroma [43, 44]. Two large international studies analyzed the treatment and prognostic factors of PPB and reported similar outcomes. The 5-year event free survival (EFS) rates in the American and European studies were 82% and 83.3%, respectively, while the 5-year overall survival (OS) rate was 91% in both studies [44, 45]. Type II and III PPB seemed to have a poorer prognosis. Bisogno et al. showed a 5-year EFS rate of up to 42.9% and a 5-year OS rate of 57.2%, with no difference between types II and III [46]. Messinger et al. reported that the 5-year EFS rates of patients with type II and type III, were 59% and 37%, respectively, while the 5-year OS rates were 71% and 53%, respectively [46]. The extent of tumor resection at the diagnosis, tumor invasiveness, and parietal pleural involvement were identified as prognostic factors [45]. The prognosis was not significantly influenced by age, sex, chemotherapy or radiotherapy, country, or tumor size in terms of prognosis [45]. The DICER1 mutation status did not seem to be associated with the outcome [46].

In 2017, Leblanc et al. reviewed the published literature on CPAM management to investigate whether pulmonary lesions were detected during pregnancy or after birth, the current indications for surgery or surveillance and the potential for evolution to pleuropulmonary blastoma [47].

Patients with bilateral CPAM with extensive lung involvement are mostly managed with conservative treatment, as surgery is risky and difficult [48]. However, due to the risk of malignant transformation and recurrent respiratory infections, in most cases, surgical resection is recommended at the time of diagnosis for the definitive treatment of symptomatic CPAM. In the pediatric population, surgical resection of all cystic lung lesions is generally recommended to prevent complications that may lead to more complex operations later, and for identifying occult malignancies that were not identified preoperatively [41, 49]. Resected specimens should always be carefully examined for occult malignancies [49].

The long-term follow-up of CCAM is important when surgical intervention is performed. Careful follow-up is also necessary for CCAM cases in which surgical intervention is difficult and in asymptomatic CCAM cases.

## References


1. Stocker JT. Cystic lung disease in infants and children. Fetal Pediatr Pathol. 2009;28:155–84.
2. Adzick NS, Harrison MR, Crombleholme TM, et al. Fetal lung lesions: management and outcome. Am J Obstet Gynecol. 1998;179:884–9.
3. Turkyilmaz A, Aydin Y, Erdem A, Eroglu A, Karaoglanoglu N. Congenital cystic pulmonary malformations in children: our experience with 19 patients. Eur J Med. 2009;41(1):15–21.
4. Calvert JK, Boyd PA, Chamberlain PC, Said S, Lakhoo K. Outcome of antenatally suspected congenital cystic adenomatoid malformation of the lung: 10 years' experience 1991–2001. Arch Dis Child Fetal Neonatal Ed. 2006;91:F26–8.
5. Davenport M, Warne SA, Cacciaguerra S, et al. Current outcome of antenally diagnosed cystic lung disease. J Pediatr Surg. 2004;39:549–56.
6. Bunduki V, Ruano R, da Silva MM, et al. Prognostic factors associated with congenital cystic adenomatoid malformation of the lung. Prenat Diagn. 2000;20:459–64.
7. Kuroda T, Nishijima E, Maeda K, Fuchimoto Y, Hirobe S, Tazuke Y, Watanabe T, Usui N. Perinatal features of congenital cystic lung diseases: results of a nationwide multicentric study in Japan. Pediatr Surg Int. 2016;32(9):827–31.
8. Georgeson KE, Robertson DJ. Minimally invasive surgery in the neonate: review of current evidence. Semin Perinatol. 2004;28:212–20. [PubMed] [Google Scholar].
9. Vu LT, Farmer DL, Nobuhara KK, Miniati D, Lee H. Thoracoscopic versus open resection for congenital cystic adenomatoid malformations of the lung. J Pediatr Surg. 2008;43:35–9.
10. Lawal TA, Gosemann J-H, Kuebler JF, Glüer S, Ure BM. Thoracoscopy versus thoracotomy improves midterm musculoskeletal status and cosmesis in infants and children. Ann Thorac Surg. 2009;87(1):224–8.
11. Tainaka T, Uchida H, Tanaka Y, Shirota C, Yokota K, Murase N, Oshima K, Shirotsuki R, Chiba K, Hinoki A. Comparing surgical outcomes of complete thoracoscopic lobectomy for congenital cystic lung disease between neonatal and infantile patients. Nagoya J Med Sci. 2016;78(4):447–54. https://doi.org/10.18999/nagjms.78.4.447.
12. Barikbin P, Roehr CC, Wilitzkia S, Kalache K, Degenhardt P, Bührer C, Schmalisch G. Postnatal lung function in congenital cystic adenomatoid malformation of the lung. Ann Thorac Surg. 2015;99(4):1164–9.
13. Frenckner B, Freyschuss U. Pulmonary function after lobectomy for congenital lobar emphysema and congenital cystic adenomatoid malformation. A follow-up study. Scand J Thorac Cardiovasc Surg. 1982;16:293–8.
14. Keijzer R, Chiu PP, Ratjen F, Langer C. Pulmonary function after early vs late lobectomy during childhood: a preliminary study. J Pediatr Surg. 2009;44:893–5.
15. Spoel M, van de Ven KP, Tiddens HA, et al. Lung function of infants with congenital lung lesions in the first year of life. Neonatology. 2013;103:60–6.
16. Bader D, Ramos AD, Lew CD, Platzker ACG, Stabile MW, Keens TG. Childhood sequelae of infant lung disease: exercise and pulmonary function abnormalities after broncbopulmo- nary dysplasia. J Pediatr. 1987;110:693–9.
17. Blayney M, Kerem E, Whyte H, O'Brodovich H. Bronchopulmonary dysplasia: improvement in lung function between 7 and 10 years of age. J Pediatr. 1991;118(2):201–6.

18. Eber E, Zach MS. Long term sequelae of bronchopulmonary dysplasia (chronic lung disease of infancy). Thorax. 2001;56:317–23.
19. Koumbourlis AC, Motoyama EK, Mutich RL, et al. Longitudinal follow-up of lung function from childhood to adolescence in prematurely born patients with neonatal chronic lung disease. Pediatr Pulmonol. 1996;21:28–34.
20. Atkinson JB, Kitagawa H, Humphries B. Major surgical intervention during extracorporeal membrane oxygenation. J Pediatr Surg. 1992;27:1197–8.
21. Yeker R, Segura B, Saltzman D, Hess D Jr. Case report: Giant congenital pulmonary airway malformation initially managed and resected on ECMO. J Pediatr Surg Case Rep. 2016;9:43–4.
22. Jsselstijn HI, van Heijst AFJ. Long-term outcome of children treated with neonatal extracorporeal membrane oxygenation: increasing problems with increasing age. Semin Perinatol. 2014;38(2):114–21.
23. Aziz D, Langer JC, Tuuha SE, Ryan G, Ein SH, Kim PC. Perinatally diagnosed asymptomatic congenital cystic adenomatoid malformation: to resect or not? J Pediatr Surg. 2004;39:329–34.
24. Wong A, Vieten D, Singh S, Harvey JG, Holland AJ. Long-term outcome of asymptomatic patients with congenital cystic adenomatoid malformation. Pediatr Surg Int. 2009;25:479–85.
25. Ozcan C, Celik A, Ural Z, Veral A, Kandiloglu G, Balik E. Primary pulmonary rhabdomyosarcoma arising within cystic adenomatoid malformation: a case report and review of the literature. J Pediatr Surg. 2001;36:1062–5.
26. Hsieh CC, Chao AS, Chang YL, Kuo DM, Hsieh TT, Hung HT. Outcome of congenital cystic adenomatoid malformation of the lung after antenatal diagnosis. Int J Gynaecol Obstet. 2005;89:99–102.
27. Criss N, Musili N, Matusko N, Baker S, Geige JD, Kunisaki SM. Asymptomatic congenital lung malformations: is nonoperative management a viable alternative? J Pediatr Surg. 2018;53(6):1092–109.
28. Enuh HA, Arsura EL, Cohen Z, et al. A fatal case of congenital pulmonary airway malformation with aspergillosis in an adult. Int Med Case Rep J. 2014;7(1):53–6.
29. Morelli L, Piscioli I, Liccill S, Donato S, Catalucci A, Del Nonno F. Pulmonary congenital cystic adenomatoid malformation, type I, presenting as a single cyst of the middle lobe in an adult: case report. Diagn Pathol. 2007;2(1):17.
30. Patz EF Jr, Muller NL, Swensen SJ, Dodd LG. Congenital cystic adenomatoid malformation in adults: CT findings. J Comput Assist Tomogr. 1995;19(3):361–4.
31. Baral D, Adhikari B, Zaccarini D, Dongol RM, Sah B. Congenital pulmonary airway malformation in an adult male: a case report with literature review. Case Rep Pulmonol. 2015;2015:743452. https://doi.org/10.1155/2015/743452. Epub 2015 Jul 8.
32. Stanton M, Njere I, Ade-Ajayi N, Patel S, Davenport M. Systematic review and meta-analysis of the postnatal management of congenital cystic lung lesions. J Pediatr Surg. 2009;44:1027–33.
33. Fascetti-Leon F, Gobbi D, Pavia SV, et al. Sparing-lung surgery for the treatment of congenital lung malformations. J Pediatr Surg. 2013;48(7):1476–80.
34. Shupe MP, Kwon HP, Morris MJ. Spontaneous pneumothorax in a teenager with prior congenital pulmonary airway malformation. Respir Med Case Rep. 2014;11:18–21. https://doi.org/10.1016/j.rmcr.2013.03.003. eCollection 2014
35. McDonough RJ, Niven AS, Havenstrite KA. Congenital pulmonary airway malformation: a case report and review of the literature. Respir Care. 2012;57(2):302–6. https://doi.org/10.4187/respcare.00727. [PubMed] [CrossRef] [Google Scholar].
36. Baral D, Adhikari B, Zaccarini D, Dongol RM, Sah B. Congenital pulmonary airway malformation in an adult male: a case report with literature review. Case Rep Pulmonol. 2015;2015:743452.
37. Hamanaka R, Yagasaki H, Kohno M, Masuda R, Iwazaki M. Congenital cystic adenomatoid malformation in adults: report of a case presenting with a recurrent pneumothorax and a literature review of 60 cases. Respir Med Case Rep. 2019;26:328–32.
38. Laberge JM, Puligandla P, Flageole H. Asymptomatic congenital lung malformations. Semin Pediatr Surg. 2005;14:16–33.
39. Hartman GE, Shochat SJ. Primary pulmonary neoplasms of childhood: a review. Ann Thorac Surg. 1983;36:108–19.
40. Nasr A, Himidan S, Pastor AC, Taylor G, Kim PC. Is congenital cystic adenomatoid malformation a premalignant lesion for pleuropulmonary blastoma? J Pediatr Surg. 2010;45:1086–9. https://doi.org/10.1016/j.jpedsurg.2010.02.067.
41. Papagiannopoulos KA, Sheppard M, Bush AP, Goldstraw P. Pleuropulmonary blastoma: is prophylactic resection of congenital lung cysts effective? Ann Thorac Surg. 2001;72:604–5.
42. Casagrande A, Pederiva F. Association between congenital lung malformations and lung tumors in children and adults. A systematic review. J Thorac Oncol. 2016. https://doi.org/10.1016/j.jtho.2016.06.023.
43. Boman F, Hill DA, Williams GM, Chauvenet A, Fournet JC, Soglio DB, Messinger Y, Priest JR. Familial association of pleuropulmonary blastoma with cystic nephroma and other renal tumors: a report from the international pleuropulmonary blastoma registry. J Pediatr. 2006;149:850–4. https://doi.org/10.1016/j.jpeds.2006.08.068.
44. Hill DA, Ivanovich J, Priest JR, Gurnett CA, Dehner LP, Desruisseau D, Jarzembowski JA, Wikenheiser-Brokamp KA, Suarez BK, Whelan AJ, et al. DICER1 mutations in familial pleuropulmonary blastoma. Science. 2009;325:965. https://doi.org/10.1126/science.1174334.
45. Bisogno G, Brennan B, Orbach D, Stachowicz-Stencel T, Cecchetto G, Indolfi P, Bien E, Ferrari A, Dommange-Romero F. Treatment and prognostic factors in pleuropulmonary blastoma: an EXPeRT report.

Eur J Cancer Oxf Engl 1990. 2014;50:178–84. https://doi.org/10.1016/j.ejca.2013.08.015.
46. Messinger YH, Stewart DR, Priest JR, Williams GM, Schultz KA, Yang J, Doros L, Rosenberg PS, Hill DA, Dehner LP. Pleuropulmonary blastoma: a report on 350 central pathology confirmed pleuropulmonary blastoma cases by the international pleuropulmonary blastoma registry. Cancer. 2015;121:276–85. https://doi.org/10.1002/cncr.29032.
47. Leblanc C, Baron M, Desselas E, Phan MH, Rybak A, Thouvenin G, Lauby C, Irta S. Congenital pulmonary airway malformations: state-of-the-art review for pediatrician's use. Eur J Pediatr. 2017;176:1559–71.
48. Feng A, Cai H, Sun Q, Zhang Y, Chen L, Meng F. C ongenitalcysticadenomatoidmalformationoflunginad ults: 2 rare cases report and review of the literature. Diagn Pathol. 2012;7(1):37.
49. Papagiannopoulos K, Hughes S, Nicholson AG, Goldstraw P. Cystic lung lesions in the pediatric and adult population: surgical experience at the Brompton hospital. Ann Thorac Surg. 2002;73(5):1594–8.

MIX
Papier aus verantwortungsvollen Quellen
Paper from responsible sources
FSC® C105338

If you have any concerns about our products,
you can contact us on
**ProductSafety@springernature.com**

In case Publisher is established outside the EU,
the EU authorized representative is:
**Springer Nature Customer Service Center GmbH**
**Europaplatz 3, 69115 Heidelberg, Germany**

Printed by Libri Plureos GmbH
in Hamburg, Germany